safe kids, smart parents

What Parents Need to Know to
Keep Their Children Safe

REBECCA BAILEY, PH.D.

WITH ELIZABETH BAILEY, RN BC

WITH A FOREWORD BY TERRY PROBYN

simon & schuster paperbacks

NEW YORK   LONDON   TORONTO   SYDNEY   NEW DELHI

Simon & Schuster Paperbacks
1230 Avenue of the Americas
New York, NY 10020

First Simon & Schuster trade paperback edition June 2013

SIMON & SCHUSTER PAPERBACKS and colophon are
registered trademarks of Simon & Schuster, Inc.

For information about special discounts for bulk purchases,
please contact Simon & Schuster Special Sales at
1-866-506-1949 or business@simonandschuster.com

The Simon & Schuster Speakers Bureau can bring authors
to your live event. For more information or to book an event
contact the Simon & Schuster Speakers Bureau at
1-866-248-3049 or visit our website at www.simonspeakers.com.

Designed by Ruth Lee-Mui

Manufactured in the United States of America

1   3   5   7   9   10   8   6   4   2

Library of Congress Cataloging-in-Publication Data
Bailey, Rebecca Anne.
Safe kids, smart parents : what parents need to know to keep their children safe /
Rebecca Bailey, Ph.D. with Elizabeth Bailey, RN BC; introduction by Terry Probyn.
p. cm.
1. Safety education. 2. Children—Crimes against—Prevention. 3. Children—
Protection. 4. Critical thinking in children. 5. Parenting. I. Bailey, Elizabeth,
RN. II. Title.
HQ770.7.B33 2013
613.6083—dc23
2012047452

ISBN 978-1-4767-0044-1
ISBN 978-1-4767-0046-5(ebook)

contents

a mother's words

I am hoping that you will read this book and share it with your children. No one should ever go through what I endured. Perhaps something you read here will prevent a tragedy from happening.

I compare my experience with that of a combat soldier. No, I have never fought in a war, but the hostility that went on inside my mind is what I imagine a seasoned veteran experiences after years of fighting off the enemy; but I was no hero and my enemy was unknown. I was just adrift in a battlefield of lost answers for eighteen agonizing years, coping through a mental mechanism I like to call autopilot.

On June 10, 1991, my reality was shot into chaos when my beautiful, innocent baby girl was kidnapped. My enemy took away my firstborn and a would-be lifetime of memories, as well as countless other things. Life is never the same after the tragedies of war, but as human beings, we cope. I knew my life would never be the same, but through years of traditional counseling, autopilot coping, and nursing a flame of vigor that never burned out, I kept hope alive.

I suffered eighteen hellish years wondering what had happened to my daughter. As I reflect back on this real life nightmare that I could never wake from, something inside kept telling me that I would see her again, but I had no idea if it would be in this lifetime or another. And then on August 27, 2009, my baby girl, now twenty-nine years old, walked back into my life just as quickly as she had disappeared that horrific Monday morning. However, I was now faced with the challenge of how to reintegrate with not only my own daughter, but with her two daughters as well.

How do you cope with such an overwhelming shock? I hope none of you ever have to grapple with putting loved ones who have become practically strangers back together and figuring out how to live with each other. I am so grateful she is back, but it has been a very demanding and difficult task.

The first few weeks of reunification were rough for all of us. There were times when I thought that I couldn't handle all of the changes we were going through, but I also knew that in the end it would all be worth it. I knew that no matter how tough it was for all of us, I would never give up hope that we'd get through it, just like I knew I could never give up the hope of holding her in my arms again and telling her that I love her.

I have quite a bit of fear pent up inside me that doesn't necessarily show on the outside. Imagine your worst nightmare and then being forced to live it. For eighteen years of my life I was not in control of the situation—not a damn thing I could do about some jerk kidnapping my kid, no idea what had happened to my kid or where she was, and no clue as to where to even look for her, except in my mind and my soul. Later I lived in fear that it would happen again, terrified that some other ***** or maybe the same one, who knows, would take my younger daughter away from me, too. Live with that for eighteen years and it is only to be expected that fear takes over. This is the condition of simultaneously being a victim and a survivor. It is not likely any of you will have to experience this pain but if you have lost your child for even a minute you know a bit of what I am referring to.

I am so glad this book has been written. Kids need to know what to do emotionally as well as physically in scary, challenging situations. Children need tools and techniques that not only give them power, but knowledge, too, so that the risks of the worst-case scenario are greatly diminished. Think back to when you were really young. What did your parents teach you? How much did you talk to them about the really difficult topics? Abduction is scary. Abuse and exploitation are terrifying. But, please don't avoid this book. You never know when something you read or say to your child might make the difference between avoiding a difficult, scary situation or preventing a true tragedy.

—Terry Probyn

safe kids,
smart parents

directions for using
safe kids, smart parents

We think that keeping your child safe can be easy, interactive, and fun. Hopefully, after reading this book, you will feel the same way. Safety is about teaching kids to be aware of their environment and how to make safe and appropriate choices throughout their day. But children need help to develop critical thinking skills so they can make those "good" choices. We believe that whether you are establishing ground rules for safety, having a discussion about ways to avoid unsafe situations, playing games to increase awareness, or demonstrating what not to do, you are helping children avoid danger while enhancing their ability to judge and manage their world. In part, our focus is on abduction, because that's our area of expertise, but the principles apply to all situations for keeping kids safe.

To help you on your journey, we've organized this book into several different sections. The first part of *Safe Kids, Smart Parents* is directed toward adults and will give you both background on the dangers your children face and strategies for teaching your children how to navigate their world.

The second part, the Safe Kid Kit, is divided into eight sections. The Safe Kid Kit has worksheets, activities, samples, and resources. We've even included a section written just for kids. You and your child can read and work through the Safe Kid Kit together or separately in order to help make the concepts we'll discuss more clear.

Practice is repetition; that's why they say, "practice, practice, practice." When safety fundamentals become second nature, that's when you have safe kids, smart parents. The ideas in this book are meant to be easy and we want you to hear them more than once in various situations. We talk about the same ideas for kids of *different* ages and you should too!

Finally, all of the examples in this book are true. Throughout *Safe Kids, Smart Parents,* we've used stories pulled from our many years of work and family experience to help illuminate different concepts. We have changed names, dates, and locations, and have combined some stories to maintain the privacy of family members and the people we work with.

Our goal is simple: safer kids. To realize it, we have written this book so it guides you and your child through the fundamentals of safety, quickly and effortlessly. We want it to be a reference you can come back to again and again. More than anything, we hope it helps achieve your goal of safer, smarter, happier kids.

We wish you and your family success. Stay safe!!

what's this all about?

Knowledge

Communication

Love

When your children were very little did you ever take them to the beach or to a pool? Remember what it was like the first time? Most likely you set them down equipped in life preservers or Floaties and stayed right next to them as they stuck a toe in the water. Or maybe your kids are little right now and you are just getting ready to introduce them to a wading pool, buying them that preserver along with sunscreen. The next time you return to the pool they might be a year older and a year wiser, perhaps you will stand back a bit more, maybe even have a casual conversation with the person standing next to you.

As the years go on and you visit the beach or pool, most children will increase their competency and confidence near and in the water. Many will have been taught to swim. They will have been reminded repeatedly not to swim right after eating, not to swim out too far, not to run alongside the pool's edge. They've learned lessons, mastered skills. Before you know it you will pick up a magazine and finish a whole article as your child plays in the water. It's not that you don't care or worry about your child, it's just that you have begun the process of letting them grow up. They have shown you that they have the skills to handle a situation they really couldn't handle before. At some point you can even sit down and read a whole chapter undisturbed. The progression happens steadily and slowly.

why read this book?

You already know that you are a good parent. You already know your kids well. But there are some tough subjects facing kids and families these days: abduction, exploitation, abuse, social media, bullying, and survival, among others. These subjects can be hard to talk about and you may want a little help. Sometimes parents and caregivers think this "tough stuff" is too scary to talk about. But what are the facts? How do the experts tackle these subjects? In this book, we will give you the knowledge and tools to understand and talk to your kids and your family about safety; abduction, exploitation, social media, marketing, and other complex subjects facing kids today. By addressing these big subjects with your kids, you will provide them with an opportunity. This can be an opportunity for your children to learn, to practice acting like an adult while you are there to help, an opportunity for them to think things through. Just like taking them to the pool, over time they will show you that they have the skills to handle various situations. It takes time and it takes repetition, but little by little they will understand and learn.

By beginning to talk about these things when your kids are little, you are preparing them for the future. Your kids can learn to adapt to new situations safely and wisely and how to bounce back quickly from problems. By honestly addressing difficult topics, they can learn some very important critical-thinking skills, like how to analyze situations and then make good choices in response. By discussing circumstances running from the most extreme to the much less severe, you can equip your children to safely face a complicated world.

Here's my promise: You can teach your children tools and techniques to give them power in challenging situations. You can teach your children how to be strong and how to protect themselves, and you can do it without using fear or threats. And while you teach them, you will develop a closer, more trusting relationship with them, and your child will be able to understand and safely manage the bigger world.

information

Thirty-five years ago in a small town outside of Boston my sister and I had a friend who disappeared. No one talked about it. All we knew was that she was gone. We would drive by her house on the way to school and silently speculate about what had happened. I was haunted by the thought of her beautiful blond ringlets and her infectious dimples. She had been the definition of perfection in my mind.

It was not until many years later I found out that her image also haunted my older sister, Elizabeth. Comparing notes, we discovered we had very different memories of what had occurred and no way to substantiate them. What research we could do yielded no new information. No one we spoke with knew what had happened. What were the circumstances behind her disappearance? Had she ever been found? No one knew. Her story stopped with her disappearance. All we know now is what we knew then: She was just gone, or as we say now, she had "gone missing."

A few years later it happened again. A childhood camp friend disappeared. I was old enough then to remember rumors of an upsetting story, possibly a familial abduction gone awry, or maybe even the work of a serial killer, but again, there was no forthright discussion in our house or in the community. Instead, there were rumors and a silent acceptance of the girl's disappearance. Questions were not encouraged, answers not given. Perhaps it was a symptom of fear; discussing the unbelievable, the terrifying, might make it happen. But, as parents, we have a responsibility to discuss these difficult topics with our children. All kids need reliable information. Yes, of course, how you talk about tough topics differs with a child's age, but, again, all kids need information. That is just common sense.

In 1993 a sociopath career criminal took twelve-year-old Polly Klaas from her bedroom in Petaluma, California. Most of the young people in the surrounding communities were aware of what had happened. The media covered her kidnapping extensively, sharing both facts and rumors. Sifting through both, preteens and teens struggled to figure out what had occurred and what might have prevented the tragedy. Most of these young people wrestled also with overwhelming feelings of powerlessness and extreme anxiety and finally settled on an attitude of acceptance toward the unlikely and unimaginable. Surprisingly, few parents connected their child's heightened anxiety with Klaas's abduction. When, two months after her abduction, a man was arrested and confessed to killing Polly, many wanted to put the tragedy behind them. It seemed like everyone wanted to isolate the event, and deny that it might impact their own families. The reverse in fact happened: fear of talking about such a sad and scary event stifled real conversation. Many of the kids wrestled alone with their feelings.

Recently, an editorial ran in a local paper written by a young woman still living in the community from which Polly Klaas was abducted. This young woman recently learned all the facts surrounding Polly's disappearance. She writes that, despite all the time that has passed, it was useful for her to learn the facts surrounding Polly's disappearance because it clarified some of her parents' protective behavior toward her when she was a child. She added that once she understood the roots of her parents' fear she was finally able to make sense of her own fear of the dark. Why did she have to wait until adulthood, however, to learn the truth? She wisely suggests that children need age-appropriate information about significant events in their neighborhoods to help them understand their parents' actions and reactions.

knowledge

Children need to have an accurate understanding of the events that directly impact their community and the adults around them. Sometimes parents and adult caregivers struggle with how to explain complex and frightening events to children. Most parents struggled with what to say after the terrorist attacks of 9/11. What was too much, and what was too little? What would help, what might harm? Most of us concluded that something had to be said so that children could understand the shell-shocked faces of their parents and the adults they interacted with. Knowledge, the right sort explained in the right way, was essential to help kids of all ages deal with the facts and images of that shocking day. Helping parents and kids talk about uncomfortable topics—from abduction, sexual abuse, and exploitation to shocking events, whether local or international—is a goal of this book. And that begins with . . .

communication

Sixteen years later, a young woman named Jaycee Lee Dugard ended up in my care. She is a survivor of an abduction that lasted eighteen years. We have spent hours of work together trying to sort out what it took for her to survive her experience. We have reached the conclusion that no one can truly predict the outcome of these tragic situations. But the subject must not be avoided. Parents need to talk with their children in an honest and appropriate manner. They need to find ways to communicate facts, concerns, inevitable uncertainties, and ways to deal with them. Children, too, need to give voice to their fears, to be provided with reassurance, and to learn how to find answers to their questions. As is true for most important topics relating to children, parents can't avoid talking about them just because it is difficult. Indeed, a parent's willingness to communicate openly and to revisit a tough topic as often as necessary is the first step in making such talks less difficult. As this book will explain, the most important part of communication is to look and listen to what *you* are communicating even as you look and listen to what your child is communicating back to you.

love

Love and the skills of communication are the gifts you can give to your child by showing them the way you deal with these frightening, overwhelming, and unimaginable subjects. Managing the feelings, the discussion, and the actions surrounding subjects like abduction will provide them with tools they can carry into life. These tools can make the worst-case scenario less likely; they can help a frightened kid be a little less scared, an uncertain child more confident. The most powerful weapon with which you can arm your child is the certainty of your love, and preparing your child to confront the world safely is just one of the many ways you can convey that love. Which is why my sister and I firmly believe that addressing these difficult topics in creative, empowering ways might be the most important conversations, and the most meaningful, you and your children have.

two

don't be afraid

The best ways to protect your children are to:
encourage discussion, and
empower through knowledge.

Mention abduction or exploitation of a child to anyone and you will get a strong reaction. It is horrific, unsettling, and, most conclude, something that could never happen to their children or their loved ones. And yet it seems that it's all around us. A popular coach is found guilty of molestation. A man confesses to the abduction and murder of a child. The unfolding stories are broadcast in the news and in the headlines, on the cover of magazines visible in the checkout line at the supermarket. The numbers in news reports and sound bites are confusing and frightening. You might have heard that 800,000 children are reported "missing" each year. You might have heard about 58,000 family abductions. You might have heard that a larger number of children are kidnapped every year. What is the truth? How scared should we be? We all know that one report of a missing or abducted child is one too many! Deciphering and interpreting the numbers are best left to the experts; we must keep our kids safe regardless.

It might help you to know what the reality is. Those big numbers are *reports* of missing children: this includes runaways and kids who are missing temporarily; it can even include kids who are late for a custody drop-off. Sometimes missing persons are listed more than one time in the database, and all of the statistics available are based on reports by the Department of Justice.

The fact is that abduction by a stranger is rare. The numbers may relate to all kinds of situations and may not be accurate. So let's not focus on the numbers. Let's focus on our children's safety and well-being.

The Truth About Abduction

- 797,500 children younger than eighteen were reported missing during a one-year period in a recent study from the Department of Justice.
- 203,900 children were the victims of family abductions.
- 58,200 children were the victims of nonfamily abductions.
- 115 children were the victims of "stereotypical" kidnapping.

why we are afraid

When lighted billboards on the highway announce the latest child taken—red alert, keep eyes peeled, a child has been taken!—many of us make note of the wanted car model and license plate. We silently commit ourselves to spotting the car and bringing the child home. Others ignore it all, hoping their children in the backseat have not seen the billboard, the news flash, the magazine headline, and therefore will not be as frightened as we are.

We are afraid for our children's sake. Makes sense, doesn't it? It is so hard to know if it is better to educate our kids or just let them stay innocent about the world around them. Or perhaps we conclude we must educate them, but not too soon, not when they're so young. Odds are that someone asks, "And what is the reality? How many children go missing every day? How many of those have been kidnapped?" But does the number really matter? Even one missing child seems unacceptable. Perhaps a friend will exclaim, "How can frightening the kids teach them to be smart and how to make good choices?" But how can leaving something unaddressed or unacknowledged prepare anyone for what they hear, see, or experience?

As much as some parents might like to, you can't sit on your kids' shoulders ready to jump in with your opinion whenever they're about to make a risky choice. What you hope is that they've listened enough through the years to make decisions that should keep them from harm, but as they grow older it becomes up to them.

When they were babies they seemed so pure, so perfect, and so under our control. What happened? When did you lose your ability to keep the world from harming them? Or did you? How do you teach your children common sense in this very complicated world? And how do you talk to them about scary things like abduction without making them afraid?

encouraging discussion

But what, you ask, does *encouraging discussion* mean? What should you tell your child about abduction or other scary subjects? What is it that they need to know? The truth is that it depends. Children differ tremendously, by temperament and maturity, and *when* you should talk to your children and *how much* you should tell them are best judged by you, of course. But a good starting point for every discussion is the truth that abductions do not happen very often. Before you hear that and conclude ignorance really is bliss, realize that chances are your children—no matter their age—have heard something about abduction and exploitation somewhere and need to talk about it.

Talking About Abduction
- Consider your child's developmental age, and focus on teaching and reassurance.

- Lay down the ground rules for safety and explain why those rules are important.
- Reassure all children that abductions are rare.
- Ask if they've seen or heard any scary news on TV, the computer, or from their friends.
- Talk about what they've heard.
- Reassure your child with the facts.
- Admit what you don't know rather than make things up.
- Encourage questions.

High-profile cases are in the news. Children may hear about them on the radio, via the Internet, from the person taking care of them, or from another child. Be aware: Your child may have heard more about a high-profile kidnapping than you think, and may need you to help them understand what they have heard. Disturbing news about abductions can come from more places than you can imagine. Sometimes it seems like news is "in the air"! In many houses the TV is on all the time as background noise and children consequently hear all manner of breaking news stories. Older brothers and sisters, friends, or even tabloid headlines at the supermarket can carry unintended information to children. Be aware of what a child may be learning when these events are in the news. Be aware that what your child has heard might not be accurate and remember that it is easy for a child to misinterpret stories and information.

Where Children Get Their News:

- From each other
- The radio in the car
- Tabloid headlines at the store
- AMBER Alerts posted on the highway
- From teachers in school
- From well-meaning adults
- From Internet search engine headlines

For example, take the notion of abductions by a family member—more numerous than abductions by nonfamily. These can be just as frightening to a child; for many children the idea that a family member could hurt them or their siblings is very distressing. This sort of abduction can also be very hard to discuss. With which family member do you raise it? How do you even start such a conversation?

We will try to answer all of these questions and more in the coming chapters, but the most important thing to remember is that your child cannot be hurt by talk or by information. Fear is not the goal. The goal is: reassurance of safety, accurate information, and help with processing an often confusing and frightening subject.

knowledge is power

So why do parents shy away from discussing difficult and uncomfortable topics with their kids? Often it is because parents don't know the facts and feel like they are on shaky ground. So, afraid of sounding like they don't know what they are talking about, they say nothing. This is a mistake. If you don't present what you know to your kids, I promise you that your kids are going to get their facts elsewhere and from a less reliable source. There's another common reason parents don't broach the subject: They feel that if they talk about abduction, they will somehow make it happen. Talking about something difficult often makes it seem more real, so they avoid the subject. This, too, is a mistake.

Here's a secret: Knowledge is power, and becoming knowledgeable is empowering.

It isn't just that you aren't doing your children any favors by avoiding these topics. You are also missing an opportunity to teach them what you have learned about the world and how to confront it with confidence. Not only will you miss out on an opportunity to teach skills that can help them feel safer, but, worse, you will also miss an opportunity to express how much you love and care about them.

This story from my childhood comes to mind: When I was young I loved to ice skate. There were ponds and lakes all over the town where I grew up. It was a Sunday afternoon ritual to skate around on a frozen pond. My mother was always there but let me skate out of sight, allowing me to experience a few true moments of freedom. However, from the time I was very young I was taught to assess and recognize unsafe conditions in the ice. I learned to skate far away from the stream that flowed into the pond and to look for cracks, breaks, and holes in the ice: I was taught to stay away from light gray or black areas where the ice might be thin. My mother guided me away from unsafe pockets when I was young, but in time her guidance taught me to assess and think for myself. At first, she kept me close by her side; in time I learned how to keep myself safe without her.

Talking about abduction is the first step in helping your children to understand it. Remaining calm and being accurate about the facts will counteract what they hear and see in the media and from their friends. Don't know the facts? Don't worry. Admit it, and, as appropriate given a child's age, go about learning the facts. The best antidote to fear is knowledge, and the best way to spread what you know—and fill in what you don't—is thoughtful discussion of the issues. Engaging our children in that discussion can help both children and parents to feel strong and safe.

the facts about abduction

The three types of abduction are:
>   abduction by a family member;
>
>   abduction by a nonfamily member known to the child or
>   family; and
>
>   atypical abduction by a complete stranger.

It will help you to be able to talk about abduction if you know something about abduction. So let's get some facts straight, starting with identifying the three types of abduction.

abduction by a family member

Here is what you need to know: Abductions by a family member are the most common, usually occur in the context of a divorce, and can potentially harm a child as much as any other type of abduction. The last point is worth underscoring. Just because a child has been abducted by a parent or grandparent doesn't mean there is no harm done, or no law broken. In my practice, I hear about family member abductions all the time, often involving custody disputes. Sometimes a parent fails to bring the kids home at the regularly scheduled time (yes, being late to a custodial drop-off can cause many complications and might even be counted as a family abduction). Sometimes a parent abducts a child in the sincere belief she is acting in the best interest of the child. Often, frustration and even extreme rage cloud everyone's judgment. As divorces have become more common, and almost always entail some level of anger and hurt, children get caught in the middle. This is why the vast majority of children reported missing each year are victims of family abduction.

In my practice I work with many families who are coping with divorce and I have found that it can be helpful when both parents focus on the emotional and physical safety of the child. When they do, they may be able to work together and more positively for their child. Of course, arriving at a consensus can take time and hard work. High-conflict divorces are by definition difficult and frustrating. Sometimes there are more serious issues, like a history of domestic violence or a parent's mental health problems, that must be considered. The right thing to do is rarely cut and dry.

A whole industry has popped up around divorce cases in an attempt to stop the damage inflicted on children by the parents who are fighting over them. Courts and attorneys, sometimes the police and family services, become involved in the hardest cases but often only after the anger and frustration are already out of control. Desperate parents often respond in desperate ways and are rarely in a position to judge the collateral damage they inflict.

Deputy District Attorney Pam Grossman of Ventura County, CA, makes this point bluntly: "Parental abduction is flat-out child abuse. The child is not property. When someone abducts their child, especially for a longer period of time, the emotional harm that's created for the child is lifelong." The parent left behind who recognizes his part in fueling the other parent's anger often feels a terrible sense of guilt. So, too, can the parent who watches the abducted child react with fear and uncertainty to what is happening to them. Let's just say that for the victim and the family left behind, there is little to no difference if the person who abducted a child was a family member or a stranger.

Time and again I have learned that people have a hard time

wrapping their head around this idea. The same was once true for me, too. I have only a vague memory of the first time I heard familial abductions defined as one parent taking the child and keeping him or her from the other parent. At the time the word *abduction* wasn't even used; we just called it kidnapping, which made it all the odder. Like most of us still, I had been living with the idea that kidnappings were carried out by "really bad strangers." I imagined kidnappers as dangerous criminals you could easily pick out of a police lineup. They were not your parents, or your friends' parents. That way of thinking makes it all the harder to talk about this most common form of abduction. The girl who lived down the street who disappeared when I was young was just "gone." In 1979 no one talked about it. As mentioned earlier, I'm still not sure what happened, but just going by statistics, odds are she was taken by a family member.

The first time the idea of a parent kidnapping his own child popped into my consciousness was in a small Mexican town I was visiting with my family on a vacation. One day a very handsome young man and his rather weathered father sat down across from my friend Linda, who had joined us on our vacation, and me at the local *taquería*. It seemed obvious they were father and son as they both had classically chiseled chins and sandy brown hair. Perhaps they stood out because of how they looked. Think Robert Redford sitting with Brad Pitt thirty years ago. The boy turned to Linda and began to ask her all sorts of questions about where she was from. I was across the table and observed a look of annoyance on his father's face. He leaned forward and told his son "finish up, it's time to go." I remember thinking how strange that was. The young man took one more mouthful and stood up. He acted so quickly and obediently for a boy his age, and he hadn't even finished eating.

It all seemed rather odd to Linda, too, and after they had walked away she and I giggled over made-up notions that would explain their behavior. The most outlandish thing we could imagine was perhaps we'd misjudged their relationship, perhaps they were

not related at all and there was something romantic going on between them. Abduction never crossed our minds and we forgot all
about them.

A few days later, we were walking through a market and spotted
them over by a table heaped with every type of chili pepper imagin-
able. The next thing we knew the boy was standing next to us. He
told us he only had a few minutes to talk. His story spilled out. He'd
come down to the town with his father four years before. He said
that his father was smuggling pot back to the States to make some
quick cash. The boy had not seen his mother since he had left Texas,
and his father had told him that his mother was so angry that she
would never want to see him again. I asked him how he knew that
for sure and he laughed at me, saying it didn't really matter because
he would never be able to find out. He added: "My dad will make
sure of that."

Linda and I looked at each other and then one of us asked out
loud: "He kidnapped you?" Before he could really answer, he was
gone. And while Linda and I initially giggled at such a silly idea,
later we talked seriously about how our new friend had been taken
from his mom. It seemed really sad and really permanent. We found
it almost impossible to comprehend. We had never heard of such a
thing, and didn't understand why anyone would kidnap their own
child. Though we stayed in Mexico for several weeks after that, and
though we thought about the boy and kept a lookout for him, neither of us saw either of them again. Nor did we mention it to my
folks. It all seemed so fantastical.

Sadly, I now know that these types of stories are more common
and law enforcement is becoming increasingly aware of and able to
deal with them. Parents *do* take kids out of the country illegally. Actually, international abduction rates are increasing, but many cases
go unreported because they often involve undocumented residents
who fear getting into trouble if they make a report.

We'd like to think that safeguards such as requiring the signature of both parents on a child's passport helps, but for a determined parent it's usually possible to find ways around the rules. Like we said, desperate parents commit desperate acts. Sometimes the court gives a parent permission to leave the country with a child and then that parent doesn't bring the child back as he had agreed to.

Once in a foreign country, bringing a kidnapped child back home can be very tough. Sorting things out can take time and patience and, often, enormous sums of money to pay for lawyers, local court fees, and even private detectives. Fortunately, there is something called the Hague Convention on the Civil Aspects of International Child Abduction, of which there are currently seventy-two member states including the United States and sixty-nine other contracting states around the world. This treaty allows countries to work together to return abducted children to their home country. It can also assist a parent victimized by international child abduction, regardless of residency status.

In the United States, children can disappear across state lines without much trouble. Local law enforcement agencies will take reports and enter names and descriptions of abducted children into the National Crime Information Center. They can issue AMBER Alerts and can refer parents to the local child abduction office for help. But the fact of the matter is, it remains very easy for a parent and a scared and confused child to pass unnoticed. This point was recently brought home by the experience of a man I know who had retrieved his child in a very dramatic fashion from another country. He then flew from New York to Los Angeles with his nine-year-old son. After all that had happened, it shocked him that no one asked his son for ID. Given all he had done to get his child back into the country it seemed a bit silly. Is it so easy to disappear with a child right in front of people? The shocking truth is yes, it is. As many high-profile and lesser-known cases have established, these days it might be more difficult to take a child out of the country than it is to hide them here, in plain sight.

So, as a parent or a concerned adult, what do you do?

In the coming chapters, this book will give you some specific suggestions to help minimize the risk of abduction, but as I will underscore again and again, common sense can guide you most of the way. Know someone going through a divorce, perhaps one you know is contentious? Pay attention and keep your eyes and ears open. If you hear a parent talking about moving far away, then tell the other parent, clue someone in at their kids' school, and, most importantly, trust your gut. Kids are in a much tougher position; how can they know what to do or where to go with their concerns? How can they say something without getting themselves or their parent into trouble? Asking a scared kid to bear the burden of assessing their parents' motives and actions is, simply put, unfair. The answer lies with the adults surrounding them. If adults are keeping a watchful eye, perhaps they will see what is happening. Find information out before you need it by asking questions, looking things up, and talking about what you learn with your kids. Maybe by asking, you will assist a child who doesn't know how to get help on his own.

How does a parent figure out what the safety risks are from family members or evaluate if there are even any risks to begin with? First of all, the best predictor of future violence has and will most likely always be history. Have there been incidents in the past where the other parent has used brute strength or violence to change a child's behavior? Does the other parent have problems with managing his or her anger? Does that parent tend to fly off the handle and resort to hitting, slapping, or throwing things? All of us have stressors in our lives, but do you and your ex-partner have coping strategies to manage those stressors, or does the child become the object of frustration and rage? The focus should be on behaviors that evidence a pattern of violence or other unsafe behavior. If your child is coming home from visits with unexplained marks or injuries, or if one of the reasons you separated from your partner was because of violent behavior, this past history would increase the safety risks. Has the child been abducted before, or kept overnight when they were supposed to have been brought home? Have threats been made? Does your ex-partner maintain citizenship from another country and have friends or family living in that country? Is your ex making plans: selling a home, quitting a job, or talking about making a change? These could all indicate a potential risk to the child.

If you suspect your child might be at risk of abduction by their other parent, be absolutely clear to your child about who is picking them up if it's not going to be you. Make sure they understand that under NO circumstances are they to go anywhere with the other parent. This is not an uncommon way for family abductions to begin—be sure you are clear about this. Put together a packet of personal information including recent photos and as much other personal information as you can include (fingerprints, Social Security number, birth certificate). You might also want to collect pertinent information about your ex (contact information for friends and family, Social Security and driver's license numbers, bank account and credit card numbers). This is much easier to do before you may actually need it. Make sure your child knows how to contact you; if your child is young, are you certain he or she knows how to use the phone, and how to reach you or someone you both trust? Be sure that your child knows that you love them. In some cases of family abduction, the child is told that their parent is sick, in the hospital, or dead; make sure your child knows that you would not suddenly disappear and knows who would be there for them if there was a change of plans or some unforeseen circumstance.

If you have justifiable proof that an abduction by your ex is imminent and the child is in the custody of the partner in question— you can ask a judge to issue a "pickup order": an actual warrant for you to take physical custody of a child at that moment. Whatever you do, make sure that it is done legally and with the assistance of the authorities. I have seen cases where people do desperate things to protect their children; it is CRUCIAL that you work within the system no matter how frustrated you may be.

Secondly, maintaining a joint, supportive relationship is key to creating a supportive environment and for keeping a child safe. This is never easy; it takes work and persistence and sometimes biting your tongue to keep from stirring up old wrongs. Remember that the tensions of divorce often create unique stressors and keeping on top of even the basics of child safety becomes more difficult. It is also true that encouraging all parties involved to focus on those basics can, in fact, work to make dramatic and damaging behavior less likely.

abduction by a nonfamily member who is known to the child or family

The second most common abductions are committed by someone the family knows *in some way*. It might be a family friend or acquaintance or maybe someone who worked for the family once or twice. This is what happened in the case of Elizabeth Smart in Utah, who was abducted and held by a man who had worked for the family. One night in 2002, a man got into the bedroom Smart shared with her sister and, against her will, took her out of the house to a camp in the woods, where he subsequently raped her. The man was identified as Brian Mitchell.

It was reported that Brian Mitchell was clean-cut, well kept, down on his luck, and needing some help. Mitchell was hired to work occasionally in the Smarts' house, doing handyman jobs. He didn't seem like he was mentally ill, it seemed there was no reason to suspect there was anything sinister about him.

This type of abduction happens far less often than familial abductions. It involves sexual assault more often than familial abductions and is usually committed by individuals who have open access to a child. When you stop to think about it, this can include a long list of people, individuals who have some connection to the child or the family: think school coach, local handyman, bus driver, house painter, or pizza deliveryman. These are examples of people who present a familiar face to both parent and, crucially, the child, but are not really known on an intimate level. By the way, children don't think of these people as strangers. After all, they have seen them around, watched a parent let them into their home, and might even be friendly with them.

The point about nonfamily abductions is this: When people have contact with your child, be aware of what their agenda might be. More than one child has been sexually assaulted by a person who came into his or her life with what appeared to be kindhearted intentions. Yes, the vast majority of people your children interact with *do* have the right intentions. But the old adage "trust is earned" applies. The coach, neighbor, or other person who continually makes him- or herself available for rides to and from games and practices should be considered thoughtfully. As parents and caregivers, we need to ask ourselves what our motivation is for allowing an individual into our child's life, particularly when we don't know that person very well. Often the decision is made out of necessity: regular rides provided by a kind coach can make our busy lives easier. But when the decision to grant, even encourage, regular contact stems from a need for convenience it is always wise to slow down and weigh the issues of safety versus risk.

What You Need to Know About Secondary Caretakers
- What do you know about this person's background and professional history?
- What might their motives be in offering to help?
- Does this person have references?
- Is your child left alone with this person and if so, for how long?
- What are the possible benefits of widening your child's

circle of adult acquaintances to include this person's
assistance?

- What are the possible risks?
- How well do you know the person you're granting access
  to your child to, and what might you do to know them
  better?

Without question, accepting the coach's offer to drive your child
to and from practice and games will mean you are able to spend
more time at home or at work; the babysitter whose advertising flyer
showed up at the door one day might save you a bundle on Friday
night and that nice college graduate from down the street could sure
help Johnny get an A in history, but don't ignore the obvious fact
that all these situations might place your child in a vulnerable position. One way to get to know people better and to assess someone
is to ask questions. You can ask: Who else have you worked for and
do you have their number so I can call them? How long have you
been doing this and how can I verify it? What do you think about
discipline and how do you manage it? What would you do if you
were having difficulty with my child? Focusing on the potential
vulnerability of your child rather than the personal benefits will help
you think about reducing the risks to the child. Will there be other
children in the car when the coach is driving? Will there be another
adult present when Johnny is getting tutored, or can it take place
in your home when you are there? If the coach is going to be alone
with the child, will it be for an extended period of time? Do you
notice changes in the child's behavior after that night the babysitter
was there that might indicate distress? Most of all, listen to what
your kids have to say! Regardless of the convenience of a situation,
your child might have a significant concern or experience with that
person.

Most people are honest, good, hardworking, and have your
child's best interest at heart. Precisely because that is true, most

people will understand why you raise questions; they might even be relieved when you do. In most cases, you will find that you can answer questions quickly and easily. In some cases, a red flag might be raised. Act appropriately: Proceed with caution; be aware and be wise.

atypical abduction
by a complete stranger

The third type of abduction is usually called atypical abduction and is the least common. According to the Department of Justice, atypical abductions make up less than one percent of all abductions. Atypical abductions are committed by someone who is completely unknown to the victim or the family, as in the case of Jaycee Lee Dugard, who was taken by a total stranger from a street in Lake Tahoe, California, or Adam Walsh, who was abducted in Florida and subsequently murdered.

Abductions by strangers involve someone the child or the family does not know in any way. The child is held at least overnight or might be transported some distance away without the permission of the parents. Nationwide, 115 children were the victims of atypical abductions in 2010. A stranger will take a child for a variety of reasons: ransom money, sexual perversion and possession, among others. Though the least common, these cases are often the subject of immense media attention and frequently don't end well. Cases of atypical abductions can form the seeds for organizations like the National Center for Missing and Exploited Children, which had its origins in the abduction and tragic murder of Adam Walsh in 1981. In the past few years there have been a rising number of children who have been able to escape from these "stranger" abductors. Perhaps an increased awareness and programs such as Elizabeth Smart's radKIDS, a program for self-defense, are helping children see that escape is a real option.

So, how do you respond to a threat from someone you cannot know who is motivated by reasons you may never be able to understand? While you cannot eliminate the risk of atypical abductions, you can follow simple rules and guidelines to minimize it, and respond most effectively when a child is in danger. For starters, it is likely that your kids are aware of high-profile cases that have been in the media, perhaps have even discussed them with their friends, and might naturally have an exaggerated sense of how often they happen. Indeed, given the media, it is almost certain that their understanding of abduction, and atypical abduction particularly, is filled with inaccuracies. Fear can paralyze all of us and keep us from taking action; it's easy for kids (and parents) to be afraid of what they don't understand. Making your children aware of the more common forms of abduction will, in fact, help them consider the least common form. Learning the habit of quickly assessing the people you know will inform a habit of assessing people you don't and also situations that are new and awkward. Being clear about the unlikelihood of "stranger" abduction, but at the same time acknowledging its existence, is a good response to this topic. It is also a way to open up the larger topic of abduction, and knowledge and awareness are the first steps toward greater safety and security.

So now you know a little about abduction and have the resources to help you deal with it. Safety and empowerment of your children should be kept in mind when having a discussion about this subject. Remember that knowledge is power! By opening up this subject to your children, you are helping them to stay safe, to be aware, and you are giving them the keys to unlock other complicated topics that affect their lives.

four

never send a stranger

To minimize the risk of abduction:
> teach "The Basics";
> never send a stranger;
> be aware; and
> make a plan.

We live in a world of instant headlines and 24/7 news stories. Bombarded with information and demands for our attention, we often pick up on the big-type headline, the running news feed, not ever having time to learn the details and content of a story. Things happen in towns and cities we've never even heard of, and yet we take them to heart. Often it is the worst and most terrifying stories that break through the noise to command our attention. Not surprisingly, the underlying low level of stress to which we all are exposed on a daily basis can make us worry about our children's safety.

Specific programs crop up to address safety concerns. Schools teach children safety in classes and maintain rules to protect them: no one leaves without permission, all absences must be cleared, background checks are run on support staff, and video cameras are installed at strategic locations. Teachers, parents, and concerned adults make sure children are taught to "say no to drugs," never to drink and drive, not to talk to strangers, to look both ways crossing the street, and the list goes on and on.

I get it. You are concerned for your children's safety and you want to teach them everything you can to keep them out of harm's way. Often this concern becomes a list of rules to memorize. I am all for rules, checklists, and action plans, but it is worth pausing to ask: Are your children learning the skills of good communication? Are they learning how to set boundaries? Are they learning to analyze a situation and to take appropriate action? Of course, rules can help to maintain your child's safety, but so does learning to think and communicate! Help children to "think it through," to analyze a situation, and then act accordingly, and you will be providing them with the tools they need to protect themselves.

the basics

Let's talk about some safety basics. You are probably pretty knowledgeable in this area already. You know that teaching your child their full name, their home address, and phone number (whether cell phone or landline) is a must for younger children. You know that young kids might not even know their parents' names—it's just Mom or Dad to them! Many families teach kids to buckle their seat belts before the car can go, and of course you use the appropriate baby and booster seats for the younger ones. Little things like never playing around cars, never approaching unknown dogs without a grown-up present, looking both ways before crossing the street, holding a parent's hand in a crowded place: These are all safety basics that you practice every day. You most likely have your own basic safety rules depending on where you live, how you grew up, and how you learned about safety. You might have street smarts from growing up on city streets, or you might have been raised on the prairie and know a lot about safety around farm machinery. Maybe you grew up in a suburb where "nothing ever happened." The big point is you want your children to follow a set of rules that become habit and common practice. We think of them as "The Basics":

- Make a safety list of people who you and your child trust. Write their contact information (daytime and nighttime phone numbers) next to each name. In this day of click and drag photographs, try to put a photograph of the person next to their name and number, too. These are people you can call in an emergency, people you know will be there for you and your child if you need them to. Keep a copy of this list somewhere your child can get to, and make sure he knows where it is.

- Ask your child to agree (verbally and, if they're older, in writing, too) not to go anywhere, help anyone, take anything given to them, or get into a car without first telling you or the person who is taking care of them. Tell your child (repeatedly) they must do this even when they think you might get mad if they do. This is a basic rule that continues throughout childhood and even into young adulthood. If you would like a prepared written agreement, please see the Safe Kid Kit.

- Ask your child to agree not to go places alone. She should take a friend (better yet, friends) along with her. You will make exceptions as a child gets older, but generally, having someone along is a good policy.

- Explain to children that it is okay to say no if someone does something to them they don't like, or makes them uncomfortable. This is a tricky one, because younger kids have no difficulty saying no to all sorts of things they don't like—vegetables, for example. Getting the difference across will take work.

A young child I know was attending an afternoon swim class. There was a substitute teacher that day. He told the kids to start swimming from end to end of the pool. When the child said no, the teacher insisted and berated him for disobeying:

"You will never learn to swim well unless you get going!" he said.

"No," the young child said, "I can't!"

The teacher responded, "You'll never get anywhere with that attitude!"

"No," the child said again. "I can't swim. That's why I'm in swim class!"

The teacher finally understood: The boy wasn't being contrary—he really couldn't swim across the pool, he was in the wrong class. In brief: Saying no when they are uncomfortable, scared, and being asked to do something they don't like, particularly by anyone not on that safety list, is not the same as being mean or rude. It is teaching your child to stand up for himself! Encouraging self-worth and self-esteem are the keys to helping children advocate for themselves. It's worth mentioning here that children who are able to set boundaries often have learned the skill from parents who are good at setting boundaries for them. Think about that the next time you give your son a time-out for hitting his sister!

- Encourage your child to tell someone on her safety list if anything happens that makes her feel uncomfortable, unhappy, or scared. Assure her that the goal is to help her understand what happened so that together you can work to make sure it doesn't happen again. The big point is to encourage your children to communicate what's going on.

- Remind your children that they shouldn't always believe what people tell them. Children need to learn to think for themselves. Again, encouraging self-worth goes a long way toward learning this lesson. Do you remember the old saying "If everyone else jumps off a cliff, should you?"? If someone tries to convince your child that they are *supposed* to do something and the child isn't sure, don't you want them to ask you first? As they get older, children will get more confident about analyzing a situation and making good decisions, but that confidence comes from encouraging young children to learn how to think on their own and practice, practice, practice.

- Promise your children that they can call you anytime, day or night, if they are unsure, or don't feel safe with what's going on around them. You must also promise not to be angry if they need to be picked up because they are uncomfortable. Make this promise knowing full well that there will be false alarms and that when they occur you won't get mad. Those moments represent an opportunity for you to help a child better her judgment, not learn to question it. You can repeat your offer through the younger years of first friendships, the middle school years of sleepovers, and the teen years of parties and experimentation. As parents, you need to reassure your child that you will always be there no matter what.

never send a stranger

You would think the "never send a stranger" rule would be an easy one to stick to, but in today's world of dual careers, busy schedules, and multihousehold living situations, it is a lot harder than you think. Even if you're lucky enough to be there to pick a child up ninety percent of the time, it will never be one hundred percent of the time. The thing is this: Life has a way of throwing curveballs. What if you are in an accident? What if you really just could not get there to pick up your child? Or what happens when your child gets older and wants to go home with a new friend after school? What happens to your rules? So, explain to your child that you will never send a stranger to pick them up and make sure they understand what you mean by *stranger*. (Remember, many young kids think strangers are "bad guys" and that "bad guys" can be identified easily by their craggy old faces and toothless, evil smiles.) Here is where your safety list can really help. Maintaining that list—even creating individual lists for each of your children as they age—arms you with a fallback plan you and your child have agreed upon.

The more complicated your circumstances, the more important a backup plan is. Maybe you are involved in a difficult divorce or maybe someone has threatened you or your child. Maybe you are just a single parent with a crazy, shifting work schedule. I can't know your particular situation, but I do know that life has a way of up-ending the best-laid plans. Having contingency plans in place and practiced is the best way to respond to life's curveballs.

A friend whose older child was missing for an extended period of time made a code word for her youngest child. No code word = no pickup. Stapled to the child's emergency card on file at school was a note saying that under no circumstances should this child go with anyone who did not know the code word. In another case, the person picking up the child had to answer a question that was stapled to the card. Only immediate family knew the answer. A few parents I have worked with in high-conflict divorce cases have sent a "practice" person to their child's school, especially when they have not been completely confident in whatever system the school had put in place.

In one of the cases, the school released the child *twice* to the "practice" person. The child was a kindergartener who had diffi-culty remembering the code word. Mom waited nearby to swoop in calmly as the child was being sent home. Happily for the child and the school, the first two incidents had increased the school's aware-ness and it didn't happen a third time. One day the ex-husband arrived at the school, attempting to take the child home. The sec-retary checked the child's card and asked the father for the answer to the question. The father couldn't answer it and seemed unaware of the existence of the test. Sure, the father was a little irritated, but the school was alerted to a potential problem and did not release the child to the father's care.

Make sure your child's school also has copies of any relevant court orders. Be aware of potential problems, and let the school know. They want to protect your child too. Another friend of mine had a son who went to school with the children of a celebrity. It meant nothing to their son, but one day he mentioned to his dad something about the "man with the camera" across the street. It turned out that the man was a paparazzo, but he wasn't just taking shots of the celebrity's children, he was taking multiple shots of many children at the school. No one ever learned just why he was taking so many pictures, but very soon his activities were put to an end with a restraining order, thanks to the awareness of my friend's son and his willingness to communicate.

be aware, make a plan

Be aware that names—a camp's or school's or even the child's own—on the outside of backpacks, jackets, cars, sneakers, lunchboxes, and other personal items need to be carefully considered. Here in California we see a phenomenon of small cartoonlike figures on the back window of cars with the names of family members, even pets, written underneath. This could invite what salesmen call "a foot in the door": a skilled would-be perpetrator could use names and other easily read personal information as an opening to a conversation.

My sister has a nurse friend who had a vanity license plate with her name on it: "SaraJRN." The license plate holder had the name of the hospital where she worked. One night she was getting into her car when she heard a man calling "Sara. Sara. Wait!" The man rushed to the passenger door and acted like he knew her. In the dim light, she wasn't sure and didn't want to be rude, but she was brave enough to lock her doors and drive away. Later, it was discovered that several cars in the vicinity had been broken into and ransacked.

Broadcasting personal information can create opportunity for connection—this can be good or bad, so be aware.

Don't prevent your child from wearing a school coat, team jacket, or hat, but do demonstrate to them how easy it is for a person to strike up a conversation based on a false sense of familiarity. Experiment sometime with an elementary or middle school student who is wearing a recognizable school shirt or hat. Frequently, a question that begins with "Hey, my son goes to your school" can result in a child's response; a puzzled response, but still a response. Next, the conversation begins to flow. Help your child to understand that what they wear can broadcast personal information. Don't forbid the wearing of the item, just educate your child about the power of connection and a stranger's seeming ability to have psychic powers when, actually, the information is on your child's clothing for all the world to see.

The point of all this is to help your child become more aware. Having other adults aware (like teachers at a school or counselors at a camp) is a good idea, too. Often, discussing a safety plan becomes the first step in awareness. Set some ground rules and make sure your child really understands them because often adults make assumptions about what kids (at all ages) grasp that are completely wrong!

Who can your children call if they need to talk, or for help, or for a ride in an emergency? Who could help them figure out a tough situation? Who would be allowed to pick them up in an emergency? Does your child have those phone numbers? Sometimes life doesn't behave the way we hope it will; sometimes we can't change the course of events or sudden circumstances, but we can take action to keep our children safe and to optimize their chances of having a safe and happy childhood.

five

parents: know yourself

The way you act can influence your children, so:
consider how you view the world;
be conscious of messages your children receive; and
talk about safety together.

When it comes to safety, what sort of parent are you? Do you obsess over the fear that your child might get snatched? A woman I know was so preoccupied by her fear of abduction that she dressed her child the same way every day so that she could better describe him to the police if he was kidnapped. (When I heard her story, I must admit to wondering, for a minute, if I was neglectful for not doing the same.) Or are you a parent who believes in a child's right to have a "pure" childhood, one uncontaminated by adult worries over life's potential dangers?

the "pure" childhood

In my old neighborhood, down the road, there was a house where two children often played unwatched in the front yard. They appeared to be about six and eight years old. One afternoon, as I was headed down the street pushing my infant in her stroller, I saw a man talking to the kids from his car window. As I got closer to the car I heard him ask the children their names. Hearing his question, I quickly engaged the kids in a conversation. They had seen me walk by many times before and were always friendly, asking questions about my baby. Today was no different as they cooed over my daughter in her stroller. Interestingly, the man in the car didn't wait until we were done saying hello, or put whatever question he had to me. Instead, he just drove away.

After what I had just seen, I was very uncomfortable leaving the kids unattended. Granted, it could have been an innocent exchange, but the possibility that it wasn't left me uncomfortable. I felt I had to tell the children's mother what I had seen.

I knocked on the door of their home and stood for a few minutes waiting. When their mom came to the door she explained she had been in the back gardening. The house was a beautiful home that said *kid* everywhere. There were wooden toys in the corner of the living room and art supplies spread out on the coffee table. I asked her if we could speak alone for a few minutes. She looked concerned and sent the kids into the kitchen. I told her what had happened out front. She looked surprised and said thank you, but as I turned to leave, maneuvering the stroller through her house, she stopped me and told me that she had made a conscious choice to allow her children to live a life without fear. She chose to let her kids stay out front and play by themselves, and although she appreciated my concern, she felt that it was completely unwarranted. She added that the school her children attended felt strongly that all children should have the right to explore the world without the constant supervision of adults. Finally, she chastised me for jumping to conclusions without any real reason to suspect the man.

I thought about launching into a conversation about the pros and cons of her approach to raising safe kids, but this was seventeen years ago and long before I felt qualified to pull the expert card. And, it has to be admitted, her kids continued to play out front and to the best of my knowledge they made it through their teenage years without incident. But while I don't advocate dressing your child in the same clothes every day (particularly not in an age when, if you really want to, you can snap a photo with your smartphone each morning), I do think there is a glaring flaw in my former neighbor's approach: I wish she had been a little more aware of the effects her views might have on her children's safety.

assessing yourself

The goal' is for kids, as they grow older, to increasingly hone the judgment, knowledge, and behavior that will help them navigate their world safely. A good starting point for realizing that goal is to ask yourself some questions:

- When it comes to safety, what is the message you give your children about the world?
- Do you protect them from uncomfortable facts and events? Or do you encourage them to be aware of what is happening around them, both in their immediate world and in the wider world?
- Do you encourage them to ask questions and to make judgments for themselves? Or do you make sure to always point out all the scariest possibilities in hopes of frightening them into behaving as you wish them to?

I know that when it comes to drinking and driving, I tell my own children every awful story I know of in hopes that they will never drink and drive. All of which points to a bigger, more important question: Is it better to let children live in denial that bad things can and do happen, or should we instill fear in their hearts?

the parenting style quiz

Circle A, B, or C for each question and then add up the number of As, Bs, and Cs at the end.

1. **The magazine in the checkout line shows a child who has been kidnapped on the front cover. Your child asks you a question about it. You:**

a. point to the magazine and explain that this is what happens to little girls who don't hold hands with their parents in public.

b. tell her you don't know anything about it and try to distract her with something else.

c. answer her question and ask her what she thinks about the issue.

2. **It is midnight and your phone starts to ring, waking you up. It's your teenager calling to ask you to pick her up because she is too drunk to drive herself home. You:**

a. are immediately angry that she has been drinking and is underage, and tell her how upset you are that she has disobeyed you like this. After picking her up, you immediately ground her and remind her of your college roommate who died of an alcohol overdose. It's important that she remember the dangers of drinking.

b. immediately go to pick her up. You are happy that she is making friends and is responsible enough to call you before getting behind the wheel drunk. You share crazy stories of your own party years as you drive home.

c. immediately go pick her up. You are proud that she is responsible enough to call you before getting behind the wheel drunk, and you tell her as much. You use the next morning as an opportunity to talk about her decision to drink and why that was not appropriate.

3. **Your six-year-old doesn't want to wear a jacket even though it's snowing out. You:**

a. demand that he wear the jacket and tell him about the dangers of pneumonia.

b. bribe him to wear his jacket with the promise of a snowball fight.

c. question his decision and ask him why wearing a jacket might be a good idea. When he continues to refuse, you allow him to go without, carrying the jacket along with you just in case.

4. **Your fifteen-year-old plans to quit the team sport she's been playing for years. She's very good at this sport, and you were hoping she'd be able to get a college scholarship with her talent. You:**

a. tell her that "quitters never win," and remind her that she is ruining her whole life. And your life too.

b. tell her she can quit effective immediately. You will take care of selling all the expensive equipment you bought for her. You don't mind that she has nothing else planned.

c. talk to your daughter about what's going on in her life. What are her goals and her dreams? What has prompted her to want to give up the sport she has played and loved for years? You discuss, realistically, the college scholarship option and how giving up this option may affect her life.

5. **Your ten-year-old is acting like he knows what is best for everyone. One day he walks home from school by himself without telling you or anyone. You are frantic trying to find him and even call the police. When he arrives home an hour late, you:**

a. tell him his life has now ended as he has known it. From now on he will not be left alone for even one minute. You remind him that "kids are kidnapped and murdered all the time" (even though this is not true).

b. tell him what a big boy he is and how he should make judgments and decisions for himself from now on.

c. tell him that you did not know where he was and that you were afraid. You go over some of the ground rules for safety. You tell him that you love and support him but you are his parent (caregiver), and he must tell you where he is without fail. Depending on the child this can either be a warning, or have a consequence. You arrange another day for him to practice walking home with a buddy.

Mostly As
THE FIRE AND BRIMSTONE PARENT

You want your child to be safe, and because parents know best, you call all the shots. You do not tolerate disobedience, and feel uncomfortable when asked questions. When you talk about safety, you will often tell them about worst-case scenarios in order to "scare them straight" rather than engage in a long conversation. While it's fine, even good, to set strict boundaries, without allowing your children the room to grow and make mistakes, they will not be able to hone their judgment and make good decisions on their own. By teaching your children to ask you questions and talk about the world around them, they will become more comfortable asking their peers and authorities questions when they feel uncomfortable or unsafe.

Mostly Bs
THE ROSE-COLORED GLASSES PARENT

You want your child safe, but are more worried that they will be afraid. If something scary is going on in the news, you turn off the TV or hide the newspapers. You think there is no reason that your child should have to hear about abduction or abuse because it'll never happen to them. You believe your child should make their own decisions and so you give them free rein to do whatever they want. Though keeping your children free from fear and allowing them to make their own decisions are always the goals, avoiding scary topics won't help them be safe. By hiding the dangers of the world from them and pushing important issues under the rug, you are preventing your children from developing the skills to cope with the real world.

Mostly Cs

THE EVENHANDED PARENT

You believe in both safety and freedom from fear with equal measure. You value your children's ability to make their own decisions, and give them safe places to make their own mistakes. You believe that by setting wider boundaries, and talking to your children about the reasons behind those boundaries you will keep them safer and help them make smarter choices. You believe in having honest, age appropriate conversations with your children about the world around them, and that doing so will better prepare them for potential dangers. Congratulations! You're teaching your children smart decision-making skills and setting the right example to keep them smart and safe.

finding the middle ground

Of course, neither extreme is correct, and finding that middle ground that works for you and your kids starts with learning what you are and are not comfortable with, and how you see the world around you. But know this: Your view of the world can shape your child's view of it, and consequently her behavior, and this will contribute to how safely she navigates it.

Learn to be conscious of what messages your children receive, particularly from you and the other adults who care for them. If you see life as one big disappointment, your child is likely to see it the same way. An attitude of hopelessness and despair can spread through a home in the same way the odor of a dirty litterbox can; the smell is there, but goes unnoticed by everyone living in the home. To an outsider, however, the stink overpowers everything.

Think about your attitudes: Are you an optimist or a pessimist? Do you tend to view people with suspicion, or grant them the benefit of the doubt? Do you view the world and life's possibilities negatively or positively? What does this have to do with safety? Because talking about safety isn't enough; it's just the start. *How* you talk about safety is just as important.

Remember that our beliefs are set in childhood and the explanations for those beliefs are provided to us by our parents. A client of mine once spent hours sorting through her feelings about her failure as a ballet dancer. She said that her mother had always pointed out what a great dancer she could have been if only she had practiced. That she wasn't a great dancer echoed her mother's judgment that she had failed. In time, however, she realized she had never really wanted to be a dancer and, in fact, was quite pleased with her life as a veterinarian. Yet it took her years to overcome her learned negative attitudes and to untangle her mother's ambitions from her own, just as it takes years to overcome the criticisms and fears that we inherit.

On the flip side, an overly positive attitude can lead to unreal and unfair expectations of the world, and of other people, and can be a setup for failure and disappointment. Most people are kind at heart and have good intentions; but not all. Most situations will turn out okay; but not all. A child who is raised in an overprotected and unrealistically positive environment can have difficulty understanding how other people feel about anything. This child may have experienced always having things his or her own way, without encountering differences of opinion. This child may expect their own rosy view of things from everyone around them. This child is not learning how to manage ups and downs or how to assess a situation and make a wise choice. This child must "block out" reality and "push away" the viewpoints of others. This child can easily become a little tyrant who has no consideration or understanding of others, no flexibility in his thinking, and no ability to tolerate the complexities of the world. How will this child learn to find his own way or to think for himself?

I've seen more than a few children in my practice who were raised as "the center of the universe" with everything taken care of for them. They have never experienced adversity or disappointment and expect the world to continue without bumps and bruises. There is an old adage that goes "If children have nothing to overcome, they'll never be able to overcome anything." It's very true.

Sometimes the children I see in my practice have had the experience of "falling apart" when things didn't go their way. I've seen this happen when a kid didn't get into the college of his or her choice and simply couldn't handle the disappointment. Or a child will be starting a first job and will become completely overwhelmed, unsure how to proceed without constant direction from a parent. The young adult might be required to do something they don't want to do, or more likely, may have their own plan in mind (arriving for work late every time, because "I was busy"). These children have not developed any coping abilities or strategies to manage distress and adversity. They often need to be taught all over again before they are able to get on with their lives.

An important growing point for a child comes when that child understands that his parents might see things a bit differently than he does. When a child who hates spinach becomes aware that Mom loves spinach, it is a startling realization. Suddenly, the child sees himself as separate, having opinions that differ from Mom or Dad. When the child begins to understand this, he can start to find his own way, to develop his own opinions, and to develop the ability to judge for himself. This is the beginning of critical thinking and an important component to your child's safety.

By critical thinking I mean the ability to assess a situation, size up an individual, weigh choices and risks, and reach a considered decision. Young children have not yet developed these skills. Your five-year-old might believe that because he hates spinach, everyone else must hate spinach, but as your child continues to grow, you will see him learn to form his own opinions and attitudes, separate from yours (sometimes to the point of irritation). Encourage your child to do so and, with a gentle hand, guide them toward not only the right decisions, but also the way to arrive at those right decisions. Your attitude toward the development of your child's critical-thinking skills can have great effect on their learning to trust their own judgment and ultimately on making smart and safe choices.

outside influences

As I mentioned in the introduction, parents and caregivers need to realize that they are only one source of information a child receives. Families that shield their children from the events of the world can be surprised by how much information their children are getting anyway. One family protected their kindergartner from the knowledge that the World Trade Center towers had been destroyed by terrorists. There was no TV in their home and they were very careful to never discuss the "terrible news" from New York. One afternoon a plane flew over their house and the little boy responded by asking if the plane was an enemy or a good guy; obviously he had heard something somewhere. At that point the parents realized the child needed to talk with them about what he had heard and learned, in order to help him sort out a confusing and frightening story.

How conscious are you of the messages your children are receiving? Where are they getting their information, and from what sources? Pay attention to how much the news plays in your home or on your car radio: be aware of what your children take in around you.

Many years ago I encountered a woman who suffered from extreme anxiety. She reported great difficulty sleeping and had constant nightmares when she did sleep. Turning the TV off two hours before she went to bed solved the problem. The news blaring each night before she slept was fueling her anxiety and disrupting her sense of safety. In turn, her six-year-old was increasingly infected with her fear.

I was shocked when my niece, who was seven years old at the time, told me she wanted to go to the "club" for men, which she reported was near her house. Upon further investigation it turned out that she was seeing a particularly sensational billboard on her way to school every day. The billboard depicted a young lady with pouty bright red lips, and had a red banner across it that said: FOR MEN ONLY. The address was, in fact, nowhere near her house. Our later discussion, held in the simplest terms only, helped her to understand and process what she was seeing and opened the door to further conversations.

Remember, it takes two to have a conversation. Parents need to be willing to listen, and examine their own beliefs about abduction. A dear psychologist friend of mine relayed a story about attempting to discuss the topic of abduction with her husband and eleven-year-old son. Her husband, she said, got so upset that he left the room repeatedly during the conversation. The thought of losing their child was so terrifying he couldn't talk about abduction; it was easier to just deny the importance and reality of the topic. However, when their son reported hearing about a recent abduction on the news, his dad realized it was important for him to at least be present and listen to his son's fears. My friend wisely reminded her husband that it wasn't necessarily *their* child they were talking about. It made it easier for him to discuss abduction, and safety, when he stopped picturing their child. She still leads the conversations with their son, but added that her husband is now able to stay put through most of them.

Don't kid yourself. Children are paying attention and listening carefully. They are aware that kids disappear and their discomfort with the topic can far exceed that of most adults. Even a kid can figure out that it is children, people their age, who are the targets for abduction. You might not know that your children are anxious about abduction because, like my friend's husband, it is a subject they find hard to talk about. You might see it when they are playing or in the stories they tell you about monsters. An older child may show you their fear by acting like they know it all already but, believe me, they're listening. Abductions happen, and they happen to kids people know or have heard of, and parents need to be ready, willing, and able to sit down and talk about it. The topic should not be left to school-based programs, but needs to be addressed at home and at different times as your children grow.

Remember that the way you view the world very often becomes the way your children view the world; your view can shape your child's view and consequently her behavior. How you discuss any subject will change, and how you learn to listen to your children's thoughts will evolve, too, but the need for the conversation remains throughout the years.

"be alert. the world needs more lerts"

You can teach your child to be aware of potential dangers by:

playing games to encourage awareness; and

making a habit of daily conversation during dinners, car

trips, and game nights.

As you have probably figured out by now, I am big on teaching children to think critically. That means learning to assess a situation and deciding how to respond appropriately. While safety couldn't be more serious, one of the best ways to instill the habit of being safe is to approach it through play. Why? Because play encourages communication. And communication is a big component of learning to pay attention to your surroundings. This chapter offers up some tricks/games parents can use to encourage awareness and with it, critical thinking.

Of course, it all begins with good communication. Good communication is about talking to one another. Talking and listening skills are not easy to develop; they take time and energy. Practice good communication skills by having conversations with your kids on a regular basis. Start by asking questions; in fact, you can make it fun by having a different person be the moderator or question person. Some families are able to have dinner together every day, some find other times to talk. But do it! Even if it becomes one or two times a week, do it!

be a lert!

My favorite such game is teaching a child to become a Lert. A Lert, of course, doesn't really exist. It's a play on the phrase from the writer, director, and actor Woody Allen, but it provides a fun way to introduce and keep the topic of awareness alive in your home. In the course of my work with families and younger clients, I have learned any number of games—many of them will be familiar to you—that can be put to the purpose of turning children (and sometimes adults) into Lerts.

draw a lert

So, start by asking your child what a Lert might look like. One mom I knew helped her daughter draw a picture of a fuzzy caterpillar that they called a Lert. You might encourage your children to imagine it has big eyes, or many eyes, or eyes at the back of its head. This is because you want to teach children that Lerts look all around them and are aware of what, and who, is near them and what, if anything, seems out of place. And Lerts like to talk and discuss, because Lerts quickly communicate what they see and don't jump to conclusions. Encourage whatever promotes awareness without supporting fear. And remember, when you take time to listen to your child's story and ideas, you are encouraging her to be aware. Keep it fun, but encourage the child to observe and describe what she sees. And know that this isn't an exercise for just one single Saturday; you need this to become a game you come back to repeatedly.

Talking with children about abduction at any age can be a difficult task. Make it seem too scary, and kids (and not a few adults) can avoid it. Young children need to know that the world is a safe and wonderful place. At the same time, a child must also be encouraged and taught to be aware of his surroundings. A client of mine told the following story about her youngest daughter. The daughter waited patiently at the bus stop directly outside her house where the woman could see her from the kitchen window. While my client could see her daughter, her view of the road that ran in front of her house was obscured. One day her daughter re-entered the house, came into the kitchen, and told her a man in a blue car was parked up the street. The little girl said the car had been there all week and that she did not want to wait out front by herself. The mother drove the child to school and tipped off the local police. The next morning the police followed up by driving by the rural bus stop and found the man parked in his blue car. The man told the officer he was sleeping. That's the last anyone saw of him.

Perhaps he was just sleeping; maybe, even probably. But who knows? This occurred in 1973, before the flow of communication between law enforcement agencies reached the level it is at today, and before a constant barrage of media coverage ensures every attempted or realized abduction is national news before the day is out. Who knows what law enforcement might have found if they'd had the ability to look deeper into that driver's history? So perhaps a crime was prevented by the little girl's action and the police officer's follow-up. That is the power of a Lert.

The child is now a middle-aged woman. When asked what made her tell her mother about the man parked in the blue car she answered, "The car was just out of place. It didn't fit the street." Admittedly, her answer comes forty-five years after the fact, but her experience points to what can come from encouraging children to pay attention, think about their surroundings, and communicate what they see that makes them uncomfortable.

Encourage your Lerts to be aware and survey their environment. Know that awareness is like a muscle, and it can get stronger with use and exercise. And exercising it can be fun. Simple games like having a child find something that is out of place can be fun. Start with the obvious and absurd. Even a young child can identify what is out of place if you present him with a picture of a giraffe on a city street. And when teaching street-smart skills to a toddler, that's not a bad way to start. Photoshop a picture or look for wacky Internet photos. Line up three toy cars with a dinosaur on a windowsill. Draw a picture of something out of place. It's like playing hide-and-seek. The first time you might hide an object in plain sight—on top of a couch seat, or on top of a coffee table. The next time, you might make it a bit harder for a child to find. As your children get older, the game becomes harder, and they become more and more accustomed to studying their surroundings. The goal is simply to do whatever it takes to open the conversation about awareness.

i spy

Another game that encourages close observation of one's environment is I SPY: the child's parent or caregiver silently chooses an object in the room, let's say the sofa, and says: "I spy with my little eye, something that begins with S." The child or children then guess what it is and the child who guesses right gets to silently select the next object. This game encourages those same skills of studying one's environment and noticing details. It is particularly effective when you can play with several children who all compete to see who can be the most observant. Want to cut down on competition? Have one child seek an "S" (sofa) object while the other looks for a "C" (chair). Again, the big point is to get them observing, talking, and assessing.

one of these things is not like the others

A variation of this game is "what thing doesn't belong with the others." This can range from spotting the apple in a group of oranges, to using the sophisticated categorization games found easily on the Internet or in toy stores. "Which one doesn't belong" promotes awareness and rewards observation. Most children love to play these types of games, particularly when they are very young. And you don't need to explain that you have some multiple motives for playing them; just have some fun!

I can anticipate some of you objecting. "Bad guys don't always stick out," you say. This is absolutely true and is an important point to teach your children. It is also true that an individual known to the family is the next likely person to abduct or molest a child after a parent or caregiver. Learning to observe the world around them is just the starting point for children. And just as the game progresses from the easy to the difficult, from the obvious to the more subtle, so, too, will a child's powers of awareness increase. If you start with I SPY, you start with observing the familiar. If you add "One of These Things Is Not Like the Others," you include observing what is outside the norm. Eventually, these games do open up to that more serious conversation, which includes the fact that bad guys don't always stand out in obvious ways.

Playing these games isn't a means of avoiding difficult subjects, but rather ways to encourage a child to notice what is in their immediate environment and to pay attention when something does not look or feel right. Encourage children to discuss what they see, what seems off. Most of all, continue developing conversation skills. Talk and listen together. Mealtimes, car trips, and game nights are all opportunities to understand how your child thinks about safety and increase awareness. Encourage your child's awareness and abilities to communicate.

Games for Lerts!

Draw a Lert—Help make up an imaginary creature to help your child visualize awareness.

I SPY—Try to have your child guess the objects from your descriptions.

What's Missing?—Hide an object from a set, and have your child locate the missing item.

Does this Fit?—Stick a DVD case in with a pile of newspapers, or put an orange in the bowl with some apples. Ask your child to find the thing that doesn't fit in with the others.

Fill in the Blank—Mad Libs and fill in the blanks help with both grammar and awareness.

Where's Waldo? and I SPY books—These are a great way to practice reading and being a Lert together.

Find the Alphabet in Nature—Take a walk together and see how many letter shapes you can find in nature.

seven

think it through

Analyze situations using:
   the Safety Equation and
   the Safety List.

Games can help turn a child into a Lert, and the Safety List spelled out in chapter four can help an alert child think through basic safety. As your young child grows into a young adult, the simple rules behind that list—knowing who to call in an emergency, who to tell where they're going, how to respond to a stranger's requests for information or help, and when to tell a trusted adult if something strikes them as odd or threatening—will help maintain their safety. Briefly go back to chapter four, review the list on page 29, and make sure you have revisited it recently with your children. My sister's fifteen-year-old is convinced she will never encounter a problem and it's all overkill and exaggeration, but she still follows the rules her mother laid out years ago.

thinking it through

When I was twenty-two, I did a dumb thing (well, I did a lot of dumb things when I was twenty-two, but this is the one that still stands out in my memory). At the time, I adored horseback riding and had worked very hard to save enough money to buy a horse. When I finally had enough, I saw and answered an ad in the paper. When I called the number provided, a man picked up the phone and spoke knowledgeably about the horse he was selling. He explained that the horse was stabled in a fairly remote and hard-to-find area, so I agreed to meet him part of the way there. From our meeting spot, he promised to drive me out to the horse farm where I could see the horse. I hopped in my car and drove out to meet him. He seemed like a nice enough guy so, thinking about the horse I hoped to buy, I jumped into his van and off we went. To this day I remember the moment I realized the vulnerable position I'd put myself into: It was about twenty minutes into the trip and all of a sudden I realized I was in one of those vans that didn't have windows in the back, and, of course, this was in the time before cell phones. Worse, I hadn't told anyone the details of my plans. I felt the blood rush up to my face and I felt weak. What had I done? Why hadn't I thought this through?

I know now that I was very lucky that the man was just trying to sell a horse and didn't have anything else in mind. But I can say that this experience changed me forever. Thereafter, I became a more thoughtful person. I knew I had made a mistake, and I vowed I wouldn't make the same mistake again.

The lesson I learned that day and have tried to follow ever since is this: Think it through. Sometimes we are very good at understanding the consequences of our actions. Moms are particularly good at this, and can immediately visualize the worst-case scenario. When their kids are little, mothers get lots of practice: "Don't swim right after you eat—you'll drown," "Look both ways—you'll get hit by a car," "Don't talk with your mouth full—you'll choke," "Don't tip back in your chair—you'll crack your head."

Some people are not so good at visualizing consequences; many young adults are notoriously bad at this. You will often hear it said that kids in this age group don't have fully developed judgment skills yet. It's like they can't link the present with the future; they can't imagine the consequences of their actions. In fact, they really don't have the ability to make great judgments; the part of the brain used in making these sort of decisions often isn't fully developed in this age group.

The Maturing Brain

All kids develop at different speeds, but the prefrontal cortex is the part of the brain that develops last—sometimes even as late as twenty-five! The prefrontal cortex is responsible for abstract thinking and analysis. This helps explain why most teenagers and 'tweeners still have trouble with things like:

- focusing attention
- planning ahead
- considering the future and making predictions
- controlling emotions
- impulse control

This isn't true for all young adults/older teens; some are very wise and make excellent choices. But most, of course, are like me at twenty-two—lucky. Poor judgment most often doesn't lead to a terrible outcome. But the risks are too great to leave things to luck, which means perfecting our ability to think a situation through.

In an incident at a high school in Pennsylvania, a young woman called in a bomb threat three times because she really didn't want to go to school that day. This led to the evacuation of more than 1,800 people and closure of the school. The police worked quickly and were able to trace the phone calls. The young student was caught and charged with two felony counts of threats to use weapons of mass destruction, felonies of terroristic threats and causing or risking a catastrophe, and misdemeanors of false alarms to public safety agencies, recklessly endangering another person, and disorderly conduct. Making the choice to call in bomb threats to get out of school is a good example of poor judgment; this young woman was not able to think through the potential consequences of her actions, and was unable to use another strategy to cope with her own discomfort of having to go to school.

the safety equation

The trick is to be able to quickly assess a situation, and to be able to think it through to the end of the story. One useful way to approach the challenge is to think of it like an equation, what you might call the Safety Equation. If you were to turn my story of setting off to buy a horse into an equation it would come to: young girl alone + an older guy she doesn't know + a van with no windows + no one knowing the girl's whereabouts = a potentially dangerous situation. That's not to assume that something bad will happen, it just adds up to a *potentially* dangerous situation. The great thing about the Safety Equation is that the equation speaks for itself, helping to give weight to *potentially*. Subtract "van with no windows" and it's just a little bit less dangerous. Subtract "no one knowing the girl's whereabouts" and it's a good bit less dangerous. Add in "in rural area far from anyone else" and, well, you can see why I felt so stupid sitting in that van. The equation is a tool, just like for a toddler learning to be a Lert is a tool. And just as you want a younger child to learn to automatically assess their surroundings, you want them to grow up to add to that the habit of thinking situations through. A word of caution: Young children are not ready to take on a number of steps yet and should not be expected to use this tool; try simple, concrete examples of actions and their consequences like "if you don't wear your jacket, you are going to be cold," or "look both ways before you cross the street."

....
how to create the safety equation
....

It may be most appropriate for adults to make up safety equations for young children.

How do you turn a situation into an equation? Boil the situation down to the most simple, plain facts. Who, what, when, where, how is one way to think about it. Who are the players in the equation? What is the action or activity (doing/going to do)? When is this happening? Where is this happening? How is it happening? Most important, what does it add up to? Is it a potential risk, a risk, or a big risk? Or maybe it's completely safe, or mostly safe. What it adds up to is your decision, your judgment. You can make this a fun game: use it to "test" your kids, ask them to "test" you. Who can make up the wildest situations? Who can make those wild situations the safest?

There was a guy who drove the bus for my local middle school. Though he didn't have any children of his own, he was a big booster for the school, attended all the sports events, and knew most of the kids. And he always brought a camera and took pictures "for the yearbook." Some of the kids thought he was a little creepy, but everyone knew him and, besides, he worked for the school. Over time, however, he started focusing more attention on specific boys and, probably because they were embarrassed, or maybe because he targeted them for being shy, they didn't tell anyone. Eventually, however, a boy on the bus mentioned to a parent that he thought the driver was up to something odd. Then it came out that he had been investigated previously. And then it became apparent that he had been taking inappropriate photographs. But, if you "think this through," the Safety Equation would have raised enough red flags for concern. The equation would have run as follows: lonely childless male + camera + access to kids = potential problem!

The value of the Safety Equation is it gives you reason to act, not react. If adding up the equation gives you pause, discover a few more variables to add. You may learn a bus driver has an exemplary record and that the yearbook staff coordinator reviews every picture he takes of the kids. Add those to the equation and the result is much less disconcerting. Add a prior investigation and the fact that his pictures weren't making it into the yearbook, and you see a pattern you need to act on further.

We have all heard stories similar to the one concerning my kid's bus driver. Often, we hear rumors of stories. It is important that you refuse to let the sensational nature of the stories keep you in a state of fear. Refuse to convict people you don't know, especially when the stories you hear stand on only so much gossip. Rather than give in to fear or sensationalism, look for the truth first; most often, teachers and coaches are interested in your kid for legitimate reasons and usually the odd bus driver is just an odd guy. What you must do is think the stories through.

safety list + safety equation = smart parenting

Equally as important, you must teach your children to think stories and situations through. Here is where the Safety List and safety equations collide usefully. Adding items from the Safety List to the equation will always reduce the potential for danger. Did your child tell someone where she was going? How well does she, and you, know the people she is with? How well does she know her surroundings, where she is, and where she is going? How easily can she let someone know that she is okay, or that she needs help? Do the actions of an adult make her uncomfortable and did she tell a parent or trusted adult? Do your children know that they are loved? Add affirmative answers to any of these questions into any safety equation and the risks go down, the likelihood of staying safe goes up.

The more you and your children practice thinking things through, the faster everyone will learn to make a quick assessment of a situation and an informed judgment of *potential* danger. Most of us do this automatically. We wouldn't walk down a dark alley alone at night. We avoid danger without even thinking about it. But slowing down and thinking a decision through exercises and strengthens those instincts. Is there a real danger? Is it something you need to keep an eye on? Do you need to get more information or act immediately? Or is it safe? When it comes to judging the people in your children's lives: How do you know them? How did you come to trust them—did a mutual friend or local organization introduce you, or did they find your child on their own? Is your child spending periods of time with that person unsupervised by you or anyone else?

Warning Signs That May Indicate a Problem

All of these require further investigation:

- Has your child's behavior changed, or does it change after spending time with this person?
- Is your child suddenly more isolated, more depressed or angry?
- Has your child stopped eating suddenly, or stopped participating in an activity he or she always loved?

By teaching yourself and your kids how to identify these safety questions and answer them, you'll make a Lert toddler into an alert teen. Teaching your kids to follow the basic rules for safety is not a guarantee, but it certainly reduces potential risks. I listed some of those rules in chapter four, and encouraged you to add your own. Here's a brief recap:

Basic Safety Ground Rules

- Make a list of people who you and your child trust. Keep their phone numbers where your child can get them.
- Ask your child to agree not to go anywhere without telling you or the person who is taking care of them first.
- Ask your child to agree not to go places alone.
- Remind your child that it is okay to say no if someone does something to them they don't like.
- Encourage your child to tell someone on the list if a bad thing happens.
- Remind your child that they shouldn't always believe what people tell them.
- Promise your children that they can call you anytime, day or night, if they are unsure, or don't feel safe with what's going on around them. You will be there for them.
- Remind your children that you love them.

eight

protecting your kids in the digital age

To protect your kids from dangers online:
> educate yourself and your kids about online safety risks;
> keep computers and game consoles where you can see them;
> apply the Safety List to the Internet, too;
> check (cell) phone logs.

Computers and social media confront today's families with a uniquely difficult task. The speed with which technology and applications are evolving means that as parents we often find ourselves teaching our children about an online world we haven't quite grasped ourselves. And just when we think we know it all, it changes! So, what are the rules? How can you control something that is everywhere? What can go wrong? What should a concerned caregiver know about the child and social media?

but my kids don't do that!

Anyone who has children and is unaware of the presence of social media in their kids' lives is living in an isolation chamber. Typically, parents make two mistakes. Mistake One: They think that they don't need to worry about social networking until their kids are teens.

Wrong. In truth, younger and younger kids know how to manipulate a computer or tablet, know how to get online, and know where they want to go. Toddlers often learn to master the touch screens of tablets before they can even spell.

On a recent business trip, my flight was delayed for two hours. I sat at the gate and observed a child under the age of two playing with his parents' tablet computer. The child was fully engaged; quiet and focused. The parents were chatting with some other travelers and were not paying attention when their child got up and wandered over to a seat next to me. I happened to glance over and noticed that the child was playing a very violent online game, one that I suppose was accessed through the free Wi-Fi at the airport. Shortly after, the parents became alarmed when one of them noticed the child was no longer sitting next to them. They saw him within moments and snatched the tablet away when they realized what he was doing. A loud wail followed and the tablet was returned to the child, this time with a warning to stay off the game, though within a few minutes he was right back at it as the parents continued their conversation.

Mistake Two: Parents think that if they ban Internet access and prevent it from being used in their home their kids will be safe. Wrong again. Even though you might forbid your kids to have an account and lock up the laptop, kids can easily piggyback on a friend's account, swing by a cyber café or the public library, get online, and stay in the loop. Very few cannot get an account if they want one and almost all of them want one.

risks of social media

For the zillion parents whose children do have a social media account (and don't even try to memorize the names of the providers, because for every big company like Facebook or Twitter there are any number of smaller outlets for social networking online) or the parents who are being pestered to provide one, listen up: Kids get exploited, harassed, and set up on these sites, no two ways about it. They can be bullied, pressured, scared, and exposed to things we never dreamed of when we were young. The definition of *friend* has changed dramatically for our children. Go ahead and ask your teen how many friends he has on his social media account; guaranteed the number is over twenty and even as high as five hundred or more. How do cyber friends relate to abduction? you ask. Because kids need to learn to be discriminating and to recognize that their cyber "friends" are often people they really don't know at all. And that fact hasn't escaped the notice of predators, whether they're after information, money, or worse. No, this doesn't mean your child has "friended" an abductor; it does mean, however, that you must educate yourself and your children about online safety.

Let's talk about another concern. It's called "Facebook Depression." It's very real and can potentially affect any child. How can you have 450 friends and still feel like nobody knows you? How can you be the only one who has nothing to do on Friday night because nobody is online with you? Kids are very literal thinkers and are easily suggestible—"if nobody is online with me, that must mean they are all doing something great, and I'm not; I must be a worthless loser." What if no one tags your pictures? What if it looks like you were the only one who was not invited to the party and your best friend's social media page says it was the greatest party ever, with pictures posted to prove it?

Kids can take things like this very seriously. Some kids even post pictures to make other children feel bad. Social media can be perceived as a way to keep score, and your child might not think he is doing so well. For some of us, this sounds ridiculous, but find out what your child thinks. Ask them questions, engage in a discussion. Social media offers a chance for us all to feel connected, but as with anything, be aware of the limitations of the community. It can be viewed as a big scoreboard in cyberspace.

I had an eighteen-year-old client who admitted that she'd had to "take myself off" her social media website. This young woman suffered from poor self-esteem and spent most of her free time on-line comparing herself to every other "friend" who posted anything. This habit didn't cause her disabling eating disorder, but she said it certainly gave her reasons to maintain her binging and purging. An-other eighteen-year-old I know deactivated his social media account because, as he put it, "I really don't like communicating that way, it doesn't provide enough of YOU. People just look at it, compare, and judge."

Another concern is online bullying. One of the movies my daughter likes to watch over and over again is *Cyber Bully*, based on a true story in which a young teen in Missouri was driven to attempt suicide after being bullied online when people she didn't really know convinced her that she was worthless. I believe that watching the movie helps my daughter to manage the feelings brought up by the thought that online bullying could reach the point of nearly taking a child's life. She learned from the movie, but it did not change all her habits online. I had to ask her to take down some inappropriate details of her personal life that she'd posted on her home page and we had several conversations about what was true about *Cyber Bully* (notice I said that the movie was *based* on a true story) and what was not true.

How to Talk to Your Child About Cyber Bullying

- Ask your child what has upset them.
- Find out what or who is the source of that message. The message may be written by somebody other than who it appears to be from.
- Do not reply or respond to the message, but keep it so it can be used as evidence.
- If it's possible, block the sender.
- Report the message to the online service provider, to

your school (if the sender is from your school), and to the
police if there are threats, hate crimes, or photos involved.
- Visit http://www.stopbullying.gov/.

Do your children believe that something is true just because they
read it online? Just as we teach our children that what they see
on television is not "real" (yes, even so-called reality shows aren't
actually "real"), we need to take the time to evaluate our children's
understanding of what they see online. Ask them questions about
what they are watching. Do they think it's true because it's on television? Do they think it's true because it's online? This understanding of reality is often discussed in the classroom, especially when it
comes to taking information off the Internet and using it in papers.
There are many programs available to teachers so they can check
for plagiarizing. Plagiarizing is always a subject of discussion, yet it
happens frequently and often accidentally. Kids need to have a clear
understanding of where information comes from and why. Some
schools have integrated media literacy into their curriculum but it
pays to have some idea what your children think about what they
see online.

Obviously there are many risks related to social media and the
Internet. We've all heard about "sexting," bullying, picture exchange,
too much information, reality confusion, personal information
posted for all the world to see, social media depression, and on and
on. So talk about it. Talking helps your children process information
and rules. Asking questions helps them to understand. Your focus is
on safety, whether teaching them how to protect themselves in the
real world or in the cyber world.

the columbo strategy

Try talking about social media or even about the effect of all media
with your preteen. They really do believe that they know much more

about it than you do, so remember that communication is king and education is power. They may know more about the fast-developing ins and outs of the technology, but they do not grasp all the implications of social networking or even of film, television, and radio generally. You can use that to your advantage.

First, it may help to have one or more of your child's friends there and to engage everyone in the discussion. Second, use what I call the "Columbo Strategy" (after the TV detective who played dumb and fumbling to get to the bottom of things). You might start by acting like you don't really "get" it. Ask them to tell you what they think about social media websites. What's good and what's bad about them? Then listen carefully to what they have to say. When my daughter and her friends give me a general answer, I ask further questions, such as "How do I know who is really talking to me when I'm online?" "How do I know that what I read online is true?" Bring up the subject of what it means to be an online "friend." Expand the conversation and ask how much they really know or don't know about the "friends" on their friends list. Ask them if they feel competitive with one another, and if they ever feel depressed after being online. Ask them to teach you about privacy settings, what they know, and what they have used.

You won't stop the pursuit of "friend" grabbing, but you will help your child to think about how the online world is both the same as and different from the real world. And, most important, you will have opened a conversation that you can come back to over time. All this talk of "friending" and "tagging" and "liking" can seem childish, something that couldn't possibly be affecting your child, but you might be surprised. Social media offer kids a whole new way of connecting with the world, and the world a whole new way of connecting with our kids. Not surprisingly, it comes with new problems and complexities that cannot be ignored.

laying down the law about social media

It's also important to be very clear about what you expect. You are interested in your child's safety, and you are asking your child to be responsible. To that end, tell your child that you must be a "friend" on his or her social media webpage. If your child resists, you can tell them "no access, no social media account." When I told my son this he said, "Mom, if I 'friend' you, I'll feel like you are checking up on me!" I told him: "But I AM checking up on you." Which also brings a word of caution: Being a friend on your child's social media page does *not* mean that you can or should post on their page. In some cases, showing up on a kid's page is like being a great white shark at a crowded beach. The goal isn't to drive your son from the page he granted you access to, encouraging him to set up another page, somewhere else that you don't know about. Indeed, a verbal or written contract might help: what you will and will not do on his page. Just knowing you have access will have a beneficial effect. With older teens, it may help to remind them that colleges and even employers are known to look at social media pages to assess the character of a school or job applicant.

Keep the family computer in a common area in the house. While this is not a sure way to guarantee your child's cyber safety, it will act as a deterrent to unsafe behaviors and activities. Don't forget the laptops and the cell phones. It's easy for kids (adults too) to disappear into "the other room": hours can pass by before you suddenly realize you haven't seen your child around! Meanwhile, the child is surfing the Web, engaged in virtual games and conversations that most likely have nothing whatsoever to do with his or her actual life.

Also remember the game consoles and other Internet-enabled devices like e-readers. Keep them somewhere where you can see them. Maybe your kids can teach you a little about this new technology. New technology is developing regularly, so the more you know, the more you can teach them about protecting themselves.

All types of picture-sharing programs are sweeping through our kids' universe. Overwhelmingly, it is a good thing and brings joy to countless grandparents and distant friends and relations.

But remember the old game of "I'll show you mine if you show me yours"? The game is popping up again, but now the participants are a bit older and the images remain online, or in someone's cell phone, forever, sometimes spreading across the Internet. Kids are less likely to pull a shirt up or pull down their pants in a room where an adult is circling. If you are at work until early evening and your child is home alone, then talk with your child about your concerns. You might make an agreement about "no picture sharing" hours when you're not around. Education and knowledge combined with some clear rules will help your child make better decisions.

One friend of mine takes the computer keyboard with her to work if her child violates their agreement; another restricts computer time as a consequence of her kids' breaking the rules. But as more new devices arrive and technology advances, it's becoming harder and harder to dictate restrictions. Be sure your child understands that this is about safety. Social media is everywhere, and access has only become easier with each passing year. If you've had good discussions about social media, cyber safety, and you have continued to educate your children about the benefits and dangers, your child will be well prepared to make good decisions.

Safety Basics for Social Media

- Establish the rules for using social media sites.
- Keep computers and other devices in a common area.
- Turn all computers off at an appointed hour.
- Check the history log on the search engine to see where kids have been.
- Ask your child for passwords for emergency use only.
- Maintain access to your child's social media (as a "friend" or other access).

- Ask friends and family to help monitor your children's posts.
- Stay up-to-date about devices and sites (your children are great sources of information).
- Check (cell) phone logs.
- Talk about social media.

Another kind of helpful monitoring can come from cousins, friends, and extended family. Recently, when my sister was out of town with her husband, she got a call from a friend telling her that her eighteen-year-old son had posted an invitation on his social media page to "anyone who wanted to come to an open-door party" at her house. He had also posted the address. My sister made a quick phone call to her son and got the address removed and a new post added canceling the party. The local police were kind enough to drive by the house later that evening, just to be sure there was no party going on. Fortunately it was quiet. When she got back, my sister took the opportunity to explain to her son why it was a big mistake to post their home address online. Your child should be told never to post personal information such as their address, phone number, or other personal contact information online. Even the savviest kids have trouble understanding the problems this might create. Yes, personal information is available everywhere, but awareness of our need to protect our privacy can begin with a discussion about why we should not post personal information online.

Ideally, you have a strong relationship of trust with your children. Following the guidelines in this book will help strengthen those relationships. But don't let even the strongest relationship blind you to what's possible online. Whether by intent or accident, kids have little difficulty exploring online networks you cannot monitor or may not even know exist.

For example, check to see if your child is gaming online and, if so, with whom. Gaming provides the hook that some adults need to lure a child into a relationship. Your daughter could be playing a game with some old geezer who has represented himself as being her same age. In one extreme case, a client of mine had a child who was playing regularly with a group who turned out to be radical extremists. She discovered this by looking at her son's "friend" list (as one of his "friends," she was able to do this) and from there traced the group, which, it turned out, was setting up a tournament in a nearby town. Thanks to her quick thinking and due diligence, her son did not attend. Now, before I get a hundred letters from angry gamers, suffice it to say the group my client's son was playing with had deliberately misrepresented who they were and what their ideals were. The boy thought he was playing with friends in a local school district and not with twenty men he didn't know. The majority of gamers are great people, I'm sure; but this book wasn't written because of what the majority do. Furthermore, common sense tells us that thirteen-year-olds are quite impressionable and affiliating with any type of radical group of adults is likely a bad idea and certainly something a parent wants to know about.

The online world is the new megamall, stranger's car, dark alley, peer pressure group, and, yes, stunningly useful collection of knowledge, communication, services, and people all rolled up into one. What you need to ask yourself is this: Would you let your child play in a car with an older man you've never met in person? Would you let him wander through the mall by himself? What about going off somewhere she's never been before without someone she knows? What about trusting someone neither she nor you have ever met with personal information? Of course not. Learn to think about the computer just as you would a car, playground, or mall. The same safety list you apply to help keep kids safe in the real world applies to keeping them safe in the online world.

Young people easily fall prey to the interests of helpful, highly attentive friends. Not a huge surprise, often harmless, but sometimes alarming. What is the solution? We already talked about taking the computer keyboard with you if your child breaks the rules, and about keeping computers and other devices where you can see what is going on. But perhaps those ideas seems like overkill to you and, besides, your child can access the Internet through their phone or other device. Hmm, think about the wisdom of granting Internet access on a child's phone. Another place for a child to feel connected, another place to access social media. Is it really necessary? And just because everyone else has it (they don't, though that's what you'll be told), does it mean that your child must have it as well? There is nothing wrong in declaring a phone as being a way for your child to keep in touch with you and not a full-service, free-standing computer. Indeed, providing your child with a full-service smartphone should be a privilege earned only after they have clearly and repeatedly demonstrated the maturity to handle the responsibilities that go along with it.

This is not to say computers and cell phones are not useful. In many ways they can keep the communication lines flowing between a sullen teen and a persistent parent. One mom I know texts her son even when he is two rooms away. He tends to answer more quickly and with less attitude. A teen who has a difficult time expressing her feelings may do better typing them out for you. Computers and cell phones can also save time and money, and can help us communicate more clearly. "In the park by the tree, leaving in five. Plse hurry," often proves more effective than the lengthy phone conversation about why your child needs to hurry. And these days most kids cannot even begin to do their homework without access to an Internet-enabled computer.

communicating about communication

To be absolutely clear: I am not antitechnology. Without question, the Internet is a positive addition to our daily lives, but it does leave us with new challenges and new choices. It's all pretty new and sometimes we have to really think about what is right, both ethically and for an individual parent and child. Just the other day I was speaking with a well-known liberal commentator for a large TV news organization. We were discussing the nauseating, challenging, frustrating task of raising teenagers in today's world. He told me about a recent conversation, which had taken place on the set of one of the station's news shows regarding the installation of GPS devices in teenagers' cars and about monitoring kids' text messages. He was, he said, convinced that in this day and age, it was the way to go. He paid his kids' bills, he reasoned, and doing this, with or without their knowledge, made perfect sense to him.

Tracking a person's movements? Monitoring their messages? This sounded more like Big Brother than the ideas of a well-known liberal TV commentator. But, as he continued to speak, I felt a sense of relief. He was just another concerned parent trying to stay connected, and at the same time trying to stay one step ahead of his teenager. Maybe, just maybe, following kids via a GPS chip placed under their car is a good idea, and maybe, just maybe, privately reading their text messages to better know who they're in conversation with and what they're up to might be helpful. But, honestly, is that really making a connection with your kids? Safety and awareness are just two legs of a three-legged stool, and the metaphor speaks for itself. Take away communication and the whole thing tips over. Yes, you may have very unique and special circumstances. But in almost every case, being responsible parents means facing the challenge of actually discussing difficult subjects with your kids and, particularly when those kids are older, coming to mutually agreed on terms.

There are real risks in not confronting safety through open communication. Isolation, anxiety, and depression can propel a child to seek the solace of a stranger. You are more likely to pick up on such signals if you routinely talk about the risks. Yes, technology increasingly allows you to monitor your children, but this is an invitation to evasion and distrust. Even in the rare cases when it makes sense to closely monitor a child, it also makes sense to tell them that you're going to do so. In our experience, making your expectations clear, and following through, is the best way to go.

Who knows the most about what your child is doing online and with whom? Your child. Rather than try to get around that fact, use it. Educating them about the reality of online relationships in social media or in gaming is the best way to help alert them to the risks and ways of protecting themselves. Help them to see. Help them to question. Ask your child how they know who they are really talking to. Ask them what it means to be in a relationship that exists only on the computer, online. There may be benefits that you haven't even thought of, but they may also be divulging too much personal information.

If your child is showing strong signs of isolating from live humans, do not accept their interacting with people online as a substitute. Consider seeking professional help or look for ways to encourage them to connect with others.

Help your child connect to others by encouraging them to

- be themselves;
- pay attention to others;
- offer help;
- join in;
- be persistent;
- be memorable (in a good way!).

Most importantly, educate yourself about who they talk to and who they game with via the Internet. Kids need to know you are there and are aware, and they need to know you are truly watching out for them, no matter their age. Kids who feel alone and unwatched are more vulnerable: They are both more likely to reach out to strangers, and more likely to misjudge a stranger's intentions. Slow down, be aware . . . pay attention. Keep your eyes open.

Warning Signs for Internet and Social Media Stress

- isolation from friends and family;
- loss of interest in life, or in things previously enjoyed;
- change in behavior;
- recent weight loss or gain;
- increased sleep or decreased sleep;
- increased or unusual amount of time spent online;
- unusual restlessness or difficulty concentrating.

An interesting experiment for the whole family is to shut the Internet down for a day or two. How dependent is everyone on the Internet? How dependent are you on the Internet? What happens to your day and how you interact with everyone around you if you cut the online cord for twenty-four hours? Some people have tried this and like it so much that they make a practice of having a "technology-free" day once a week.

What I am pushing in this book are safety, awareness, and communication. Those words can be scrambled any which way, but they still pop up together. Talk with your child and communicate your concerns; maybe you will both learn something. Educate them about some of the things you know about new and emerging technology, and ask them to tell you what they know and to respond to some of your worries. If you don't understand a new service, application, or device, ask them to teach you about it. Let them know you are aware and watching. Feeling loved, safe, and cared for is positive reinforcement (though they probably won't admit this). That is no less true in the virtual world than in the real world.

is this exploitation or do you really like me?

To protect your child from exploitation, consider:

what is exploitation?;

knowledge is power;

self-esteem, and your child's safety.

how do you define *exploitation*?

When we think about exploitation of kids most of us immediately think of sexual exploitation. But there are many ways that children are treated unfairly. They can be taken advantage of by employers, by advertisers, by politicians, school administrators, or even by parents, particularly those going through a divorce or other big stressors. There are two things you must keep in mind about exploitation of children: First, it happens in degrees; it can range from the mildest to the most severe forms. It can be about sex, but consider the bigger picture, which can include all types of exploitation. Second, because exploitation ranges across a wide array of situations, it is important to remember that what *you* might define as exploitation, *I* might not. And what you think is exploitation—a coach demanding a child be somewhere in the wee hours of the morning to train for hours before school starts to better the team's chances—might be just fine with your child. Why is all this important? Because keeping yourself open to new ways of thinking about the exploitation of children offers another important opportunity for discussion and for your children (and you) to learn to exercise critical-thinking skills.

Let's look at two extremes. You have probably heard stories about child soldiers. In some countries, children have been recruited into armies controlled by the government, and by armies controlled by opposition groups. Most of these soldiers are between fifteen and eighteen years old, but I have read about child soldiers as young as nine and ten. Both girls and boys are used as soldiers; girls suffer a higher risk of rape, sexual harassment, and abuse. Child armies are easier to control than adult armies, easier to direct, and far cheaper to maintain.

The use of children in armies, however, makes me think about the political exploitation of children generally. I have seen young children starring in political commercials on TV for various causes and political candidates. These child actors are, of course, not child soldiers, but isn't this also a form of exploitation? There are exceptions, but most young children don't have fully formed opinions regarding our political system let alone specific legislation and probably aren't choosing to endorse or support a cause or candidate on their own. Is this exploitation too? What about other types of marketing? Is that exploitation?

In the United States, forms of child labor, including slavery, have existed throughout our history. Just like child soldiers, children were often preferred as factory workers because the factory owners viewed them as more manageable and cheaper. Children were also much less likely to join a union or strike. Nowadays, children are protected by employment laws that were established by the Fair Labor Standards Act in 1938, legislation that set federal standards for child labor. That was the first time in our country's history that minimum ages for employment and hours of work for children were regulated by federal law. They still are. You are probably aware of restrictions in your own state or city that might not allow children under a certain age to work without a special permit. In many homes, children have chores and jobs that help maintain a household. When do you think helping at home crosses the line into exploitation? Keeping a room clean is one thing. What about helping a parent run a home-based business?

sexual exploitation

Sexual exploitation of children is a serious global concern that seems to defy the preventive efforts of numerous law enforcement agencies. Worldwide, prostitution, sex tourism, and child pornography thrive. Owning, making, or distributing child pornography; luring children online for sexual acts; child sex tourism and child sexual molestation are all examples of exploitation. The definition of *sexual exploitation* also includes any situation where a child engages in sexual activities to have basic needs fulfilled, such as money, food, shelter, or when a third party is profiting from those activities. Even arranged marriages involving children under the age of eighteen, where the child has not consented, and where the child is being sexually used, are considered exploitation by the World Congress Against Commercial Sexual Exploitation of Children.

There has been a systemic and largely effective response to the sexual exploitation of children in the United States, with extensive media coverage and popular laws having been put into effect. For instance in California, Megan's Law makes information about registered sexual offenders available to the public through the Internet. Most people believe that knowledge of registered sexual offenders in their community could be a significant factor in protecting themselves and their children. The privacy rights such registration necessarily abridge are understood as more than acceptable if doing so can prevent even one incident of sexual abuse of a minor. There are numerous other laws and regulations on the books in the United States and in other countries that are intended to protect children from sexual exploitation. And the media coverage whenever a case has come to light has ensured that this subject is kept well in the public's view and has increased our awareness immeasurably.

human trafficking

The last area of exploitation I want to bring up is human trafficking, including trafficking of children. This has become a rapidly growing industry that frequently incorporates sexual exploitation. Moving people, especially kids, across national and state borders increases their vulnerability, dependence, and likelihood of mistreatment. It is hard to miss the similarity to slavery in which human beings are forced into service and often mistreated and abused. Again, I believe that information is power. A teenager who knows the facts might not be as easily led astray by a sweet-talking man promising her the moon. Most estimates say that about one million adults and kids worldwide fall victim to human trafficking each year. This includes boys, girls, and adults. In the United States, a number of gangs operate sex-trafficking rings that remain undetected by the authorities, or prove exceedingly hard to shut down.

The Facts About Trafficking

- An estimated **2.5 million people** are in forced labor (including sexual exploitation) at any given time as a result of trafficking.
- **161 countries** are reported to be affected by human trafficking by being a source, transit, or destination country.
- Trafficking affects every continent and every type of economy.

The Victims

- The majority of trafficking victims are **between eighteen and twenty-four years** of age.
- An estimated **1.2 million children** are trafficked each year.

- Many trafficking victims have at least a **middle-level education**.

The Traffickers

- Fifty-two percent of those recruiting victims are men, forty-two percent are women, and six percent are both men and women.
- In fifty-four percent of cases the recruiter was a stranger to the victim, in forty-six percent of cases the recruiter was known to the victim.
- The majority of suspects involved in the trafficking process are nationals of the country where the trafficking process is occurring.

We often think of the perpetrators as easily identifiable, but the opposite is true. The most effective traffickers may be anything but terrifying at first glance. They can be highly manipulative and can coerce their victims in a variety of ways. While the most heavy-handed methods are sometimes used—threats of violence to the victim or the victim's family can provide a powerful incentive for compliance—many victims are led into the traffickers' world by promises of love and rich opportunities for work and success. Sometimes the victim is led to believe that whatever sexual act she participated in will be used to embarrass and shame her. Sometimes victims are kept physically isolated from everyone but their captors, but all victims of trafficking are kept in circumstances where they lose control of their environment and their lives.

why kids?

What perpetrators of exploitation know is that children are uniquely vulnerable; they don't have fully developed thinking abilities yet. They tend to be more literal in their understanding of issues and promises. They don't have the life experience of most adults, and they don't have a full set of critical-thinking skills yet, or the talent to fully understand the consequences of their decisions. They are usually smaller and physically weaker than adults and are dependent on others to care for them. Weakness is the very first thing stronger perpetrators seek out and exploit.

In other places in this book we talk about the way a child's brain develops. This is relevant to exploitation because it involves the way children make decisions and how they understand situations. For instance, older teens are notorious for having poor judgment: Think about how many teens are in car accidents involving texting, even though they have been told repeatedly that this is dangerous. In another example, some kids I know jumped at an offer for "free cash," even though I knew it was a teaser ad from what turned out to be a dishonest company. It's tough for a teen to understand that there's no such thing as free money. A young client of mine was recently trying to persuade his mother to lay out five hundred dollars for a starter kit of useless household implements that the company promised was "sure to sell." The company promised that if he sold them all, they would hire him for fifteen dollars an hour (just don't read the fine print). Though all of these examples are pretty typical, most teens will continue to insist that they know better than their parents do; the problem is the judgment part of their brains is not fully developed yet, and they lack life experience. The last thing many teens want to hear is that they are being used and that they don't know it. Pointing out your teen's prior mistakes doesn't help either. All of which is why it's a good idea to begin the discussion about exploitation, and maybe instead of pointing out mistakes you can listen to what your child thinks about it.

preventing exploitation

So, is that what you do? Is that how you protect your child from exploitation in all its varying shapes and degrees? Yes. You talk about it.

You can begin by asking questions. A good time might be when you have asked them to do something around the house and they are grumbling or complaining about it. There will be a lot of gray area worthy of discussion here and not all clearly good or bad; no one can be called right or wrong for having an opinion. Thoughts have the power to form behaviors, so find out what their thoughts are. Remember, your job is to listen and encourage conversation.

How to Discuss Exploitation with Your Children

Ask your children:

- What do you think exploitation is and what does it include? (You should join in this discussion and say what you think too. If you aren't sure, look it up.)
- Do you think you are being exploited when you help around the house?
- What is the difference between chores and actual exploitation?
- Do you know kids who have been exploited? How are they being used?

You communicate, educate, listen, and engage in conversation to protect your children. Expect to be challenged, and in return challenge your children. When your children are able to verbalize their thoughts and take a stand on some of those gray areas, it strengthens valuable critical-thinking skills. When kids confront more subtle and sinister crimes of exploitation, and figure out what it all means and how to handle it, you give them tools to become more self-confident. A self-confident child armed with self-worth is more likely to resist exploitation and stand up for him- or herself. These are the qualities to encourage in your child: knowledge, self-esteem, and critical-thinking skills.

activities for building self-worth

Make a list:

- 3 things you like or appreciate about yourself;
- 3 positive memories;
- 3 greatest strengths;
- Keep this list where you can read it.

Make a collage:

- Cut pictures and words out of magazines about things you like. Paste them to a poster board to make a collage you can share or put on your wall.

Do something for someone else:

- Sometimes doing something for someone else can help you realize how valuable you are.
- Volunteer at school, at church, or visit http://www. volunteermatch.org/.

Acquire a new skill:

- Join a sport at school or learn to play a musical instrument.

Smile and breathe:

- The simple act of smiling, especially when you are feeling down or having negative thoughts about yourself, can be a good way to make you feel more positive.
- Another way to relax a little, and take a moment to restore your self-confidence is to focus on your breathing. This works well when you are stressed and feeling negative about yourself.

There are many ways that children can be exploited and many interpretations of exploitation. The point is to think it through, talk about it, and teach your children that it's okay to say no!

When Is It Okay to Say No?

- when someone is doing something that is making you uncomfortable;
- when someone is touching you in a way you don't like;
- when someone wants you to do something that's not safe;
- when someone wants you to go somewhere without telling a parent or caregiver.

You have to decide what's right for your own family but the idea is to be thoughtful, be aware, and be an advocate for your child so they will learn to be an advocate for themselves. I can promise this will be a difficult concept for a child to grasp, but if you focus on keeping your child safe from exploitation you are laying the groundwork for making thoughtful choices. If your child feels really good about herself, knows she has worth and that she is loved, she might be a little less vulnerable. If your children know they can talk to you about exploitation and abduction, they will feel a little less vulnerable. Children of all ages will benefit from boosts to their self-worth and from learning to maintain healthy boundaries. Children of all ages will benefit from learning to think things through, to use critical reasoning, and when and how to ask for help from trusted adults. Exploitation is an important subject to open a discussion about. The only mistake is remaining silent on the issue. (The subject of exploitation might be discussed with younger children when they are a bit older and able to understand complex concepts but children are never too young to develop healthy, positive self-worth and they are never too young to develop boundaries.)

Every child deserves to be protected. If information is power, why not pass it on? It all comes back to awareness and self-worth, with a little critical thinking mixed in. Kids usually don't understand that there are people who, and other entities that, might want to use them. It's up to you to help them develop good judgment, to teach them to think things through, and to turn to the right people when they are in need of help.

ten

if you don't take a cop to lunch at least say hello

Police officers help keep kids safe, so:
> check your biases in front of the kids;
> say hello to an officer;
> support, encourage, and demand a good relationship with
> law enforcement.

keep your biases in check

Police officers and other law enforcement officials often get a bad rap. Most of us encounter the police when we have, or they think we have, done something wrong. Sometimes there is a good reason for criticism, like the time a policeman yelled at a young client of mine for shoplifting and then discovered she was just putting her wallet back in her pocket. But what could have been an honest mistake was made worse when the officer told my client to get the *bleep* out of the store anyway. But for every five stories about bad police behavior, I can give you twice as many about how an officer, coming to someone's aid, was treated in an angry and rude manner by the very person he was trying to help.

What are the consequences for kids? Think about it this way: Who would you call first if your child was missing? And who would you want your child to turn to for help if he got separated from and could not find you? From an early age, children need to be encouraged to see law enforcement as friendly and helpful. Sounds easy enough but, believe it or not, the exact opposite occurs in many homes. A police officer friend of mine told me the following story: When he is in uniform and out in the community, parents frequently bring their children up to him. The first time a parent did this he eagerly greeted the child, but was surprised when the parent announced, "See this man? You better be good or else he will get you." An odd introduction to someone you want your child to go to if she is in trouble! Over the years this same interaction was noted frequently by my friend: Parents who were hoping to encourage the belief that police officers are helpful and approachable were instilling the opposite idea. Children should be taught that officers of the law are go-to people in times of crisis. Before there is any crisis, introduce your child to police officers, show your child how to say hello and how to be courteous. The result? You've just made a crisis a little less likely.

The same officer who told me the story about being introduced as someone who would keep naughty kids under control later moved to a new neighborhood. In this community parents and kids treated him differently. One kid in the new community offered to buy him a cup of coffee. Parents often introduced their children to him in a way that suggested respect. Why do you think kids in neighboring towns might have such different attitudes toward the same authority figures? The answer could have many different explanations, but the most obvious is the parents' attitude. All parents need to be aware of how they treat authority figures, particularly in front of their children. Remember, when things go wrong—your house has been robbed or your car has been stolen—the first people you will likely turn to are the police. If your child goes missing, the police would probably be your lifeline for information. Expect to be treated with respect but remember it needs to come from you as well; what you give is what you will get back.

One survivor of abduction told me that his father always referred to the police in a negative way and used negative names for them. The father used to say that with few exceptions all police officers were corrupt. The young man told me that during his captivity he never thought of the police as a possible way to get help and gain freedom.

Just as his father had, the man who abducted him constantly put down all law enforcement. The abductor made sure to tell him that the police would never help, calling them "pigs" and other demeaning names. Because he had heard the same from his father all his life, his negative view of the police was reinforced and it never occurred to him to ask them for help.

On a few occasions, the boy even saw and heard his captor talking to a police officer. The officer, of course, had no way of knowing who he was. The boy's captor was very convincing and told the officer the boy was his son. He even heard his captor going into detail about homeschooling, and his captor and the officer actually debated the merits of sending children to a local public school. Even though the officer saw and spoke with the boy, he never asked for help, or told him who he was. Most tragically, because this child was so conditioned to see the police in a negative way he never asked for help from the officer.

In another tragic case, a young man started behaving strangely after taking narcotics. His friends weren't sure what to do, but didn't want anyone to get in trouble. So, instead of calling the police for help, they took the young man home to sleep it off. He was dead when they tried to wake him in the morning. How much better it would have been if they had thought of the police as a resource instead of as an adversary.

make time to say hello

How do you encourage respect for police when the cop on the beat has all but disappeared? Seek out opportunities to interact with the police in a positive manner. Help your child see that these individuals should be respected and that they are easily approachable. Last year my daughter and I were in New York City and bumped into the same police officer three times as we wandered around, looking for a well-known bagel place. Each time he saw us he pointed us back in the right direction, even joking with us about our poor sense of direction. Our interaction with the officer stuck with both of us, but particularly with my daughter. When we got home, I heard her comment to her friends how nice the police in New York were.

building mutual respect

Now, a word to law enforcement: If you are a police officer reading this book please keep in mind how important your interactions may be to the kids and teens you meet. We all know teenagers can be tough to deal with, but they deserve respect as much as anyone else. Recently, a sheriff near my home arrived at a neighbor's house party at ten at night because of a noise complaint. I watched as he confronted the neighbor's teenage son by instantly challenging him to "get your mother out here now and shut the music down." The boy was trying to explain that it was his mother's fiftieth birthday and that she was singing her last song with the band. I observed the officer, who was clearly not listening, raise his voice and say, "You better find her or you and your friends are all going to jail." That's when I stepped forward, which did not prove very helpful. By that time, it was about confrontation, not conversation, and he treated me the same as he had the teenager, saying that until the owner of the house presented herself and the music was turned off we were all at risk of being arrested. To most of us watching this unfold, myself included, his attitude seemed a little excessive. Of course, we had not been in a car all night driving around town with him as he broke up teenage party after party and walked into scenes of unruliness and sometimes even violence. He could have handled my neighbor's party a little more subtly, but later when my family and I discussed the officer's behavior it was clear that this was not the normal behavior we usually saw from our local law enforcement.

In extreme circumstances the divide between the police and the population they serve can be so great that the police are unable to help effectively. This can pose a very serious challenge if you are trying to convince young children that the police are really a helpful presence. If this is the case in your community, begin by trying to identify a member of the force with whom you can discuss your concerns. A school police officer or high-ranking member of a local precinct is also a good choice. Sometimes there are officers whose focus is on community relations, and in one town I know, the chief even gives out his cell phone number so citizens can talk to him.

Friendly Police Activities

- Search online for activities with your local police and fire departments.
- **The National Police Athletics/Activities Leagues, Inc.,** exist to prevent juvenile crime and violence by providing civic, athletic, recreational, and educational opportunities and resources to NPAL chapters. Contact them at http://www.nationalpal.org/.
- Call your local police or fire department's nonemergency number and ask if they have any activities where kids can interact with police or firefighters.
- **Law Enforcement Exploring**, also known as **Police Explorers**, is a career-oriented program that gives young adults the opportunity to explore a career in law enforcement by working with local law enforcement agencies. It is a nonscouting subsidiary of the Boy Scouts of America. The program is for qualified teens and young adults who graduated from eighth grade and are ages fourteen through twenty-one.

No police force wants a bad rap for being antikid. Also remember that, just like families, organizations can get stuck in unhealthy interactions, but they also usually respond to feedback. If that doesn't work, make a ruckus to your elected representatives, like City Council members, Congress, or Assembly members. Be aware that respect goes both ways and be prepared to help address both ends of the problem. In one community meeting between police officers and community members the teenagers were so disrespectful that the meeting had to be stopped. Two teens called a deputy new to the area a *bleep-bleep* and went so far as to threaten his wife and kids. Rather than reprimand the boys, the other community members laughed and shouted disparaging comments at the police. Not only was nothing accomplished, but the situation was actually made worse. Ironically, it is often tragedy that brings a community together; how often might tragedy have been prevented in the first place if the community wasn't at odds and if all parties could find a way to work together with respect.

respecting authority figures doesn't mean you should never question authority

Even authorities make mistakes, so:
>   say no when something feels wrong;
>
>   trust your gut;
>
>   encourage decision making; and
>
>   set limits.

A difficult lesson for kids, particularly younger kids, to learn is: if something does not feel right, it just might not be. You have to learn to trust your gut. Children will often dismiss cautionary tales as ridiculous. They believe they can handle any situation and that they would be able to recognize someone with bad intentions. But they have very little life experience, and their innocence and youth often make it difficult for them to believe that seemingly nice people would want to do something bad to them. Of course, life would be quite scary if we believed everything we heard on TV, in the movies, from our friends, in the paper, and all around us, but kids need to develop judgment and assessment skills in order to trust their gut.

In a small Northern California town an authority figure in the community molested a group of young boys. Stories of what occurred varied from straightforward sexual molestation to bizarre stories that the man had encouraged the boys to strip naked, run around, and catch marshmallows that he would throw to them. The rumor was that some of the boys involved thought this activity was silly, ridiculous, and kind of fun, but two boys felt that there was something "a little too weird" about this game, would not participate, and told their parents about it. Of course, the game was put to an end immediately. Unfortunately, the man left the country before he could be questioned further. This story of weird, perverse behavior provided an opportunity to educate the boys and to support the use of one's gut feeling. It was also used to discourage a false sense of security: A child usually thinks, "Well, I'd never do something *that* ridiculous and I'd be able to recognize the creep for what he is." In truth, many of those who exploit children use their position of authority—from priests to coaches to older relatives—to gain mastery over kids. Kids need to learn that they can say no to something that feels wrong, and that they should learn to trust their gut.

question authority

Okay, in the preceding chapter I told you to make friends with a police officer. You should. You must also encourage your child to responsibly question authority figures. This is a hard concept to communicate, let alone to teach. All of us can support the idea that authority figures should be respected, but we need to remember that they are as human as the next guy. If you stop to think about it, what I am saying has already likely come to your attention. You get a second opinion when a doctor makes a recommendation, right? Teachers don't always come up with the right answer. Maybe you've watched some of the big shots on the local or national news who have made some really bad decisions recently. When we listen to authorities, we not only trust our gut, but we should also teach our gut. Remember the phrase "If in doubt, check it out." Encourage a discriminating response rather than blind acceptance of and obedience to authority.

Most of us teach discrimination to our kids all the time. Do you think a child needs to get a burn to understand that sometimes the stove is hot, or do you tell them, "Be careful, that's hot, it will burn" to teach them the lesson? Think first, act second. The same goes with authority figures. It is the essence of teaching discrimination.

setting boundaries

Very young children can begin to understand the notion of physical and emotional boundaries. You can encourage a child to recognize that their body is their own, and private parts are private; no one has to have their cheek pinched, and no one has to sit on another person's lap if they don't want to. This goes along with teaching children not to hit other people, to respect the boundaries of others. You can teach your child that when you are in the bathroom, they should knock and ask if they can come in before barging though the door. And when they are sitting at your desk, they can begin to understand that your books and papers, your wallet and your purse, are yours and need to be respected. This is not about having good manners. This is about understanding and respecting boundaries. If they hear you say no, they will learn to say no themselves. Teach your child that it's okay to set boundaries; it's okay to say no to sitting on Uncle Elmer's lap. The overly friendly woman in the supermarket can be politely ignored. Saying no is perfectly acceptable.

Animals are great teachers. Cats in particular can be wonderful instructors for young children. Many cats, but not all, will resist being picked up unless they are comfortable. Most often, they'll just run away and hide. But the occasional scratch and hiss also serve as reminders to children that limits can be set. Just having a cat around in the house, or visiting a friend with pets, provides an opportunity for a learning experience. In my practice I have a little dachshund mix that is most often full of affection for anyone who seriously needs it. However, if that little dog does not want to be picked up she lets out a noise somewhat like a gremlin, which backs the average adult or child away. In a few cases her warning has been ignored, which leads her to a more exuberant gremlin sound. This usually does the trick and provokes a lovely discussion on limits, boundaries, and the right to let someone know if you are uncomfortable.

But not everyone likes or can have animals in their home and boundaries can be hard to set if you are not used to setting them.

Hints for Setting Boundaries

- Be clear and follow through.
- Phrase boundaries in a positive way: "You *may* go to your friend's house when you have finished your homework" and follow through by checking homework.
- Allow your child to set simple boundaries for themselves: "Please knock before you come into my room."
- Remember that your child will feel more secure when you set clear boundaries.
- Don't set a boundary and then "let it slide this one time."

teaching instinct

How else can you teach a child to discriminate between appropriate and inappropriate behavior? Teaching kids to answer their own questions and think about the reasons behind their decisions is a wonderful way to encourage judgment and trust instincts. Making all their decisions for them never provides children with the opportunity to learn from being wrong, and constantly criticizing their judgment teaches them not to trust their own instincts. First, children need to get through the initial "why?" stage. Most two- to five-year-olds do not discriminate, and pepper you with "why?" and "why not?" Why not eat dessert before dinner, color on the walls, or use someone else's toy without asking? But once a child gets through the initial "why?" age, a parent can and should encourage and support that child to exercise their decision-making skills, along with understanding and respecting boundaries.

The first step could be to simply ask that they give their reasons for a certain decision. If it's raining don't just say "Put on your raincoat," but rather encourage their participation in the decision. Make sure they know it's raining, and then ask them what coat they want to grab. If they grab a light summer jacket, ask what might be a better choice, maybe even ask them why. Yes, this type of questioning can get annoying, and no, you do not need to do it all the time. But if done occasionally and when there is sufficient time, it can be very effective. So, too, can letting a child make certain wrong decisions. When you are fourteen and decide not to take your sweatshirt to the football game, maybe when you are freezing you will understand why your parent constantly reminded you to take something warmer. Sometimes the best lesson is learned from experience, but as a parent you can help control how risky the experience is that teaches the lesson. A fourteen-year-old learning to dress warmly can help later when that child is seventeen trying to decide whether a friend is safe to drive with or not.

Though it doesn't always feel like it, time moves quickly when raising kids so don't wait too long to start this process. Encourage your children to begin using their own judgment whenever possible. Many years ago a teenager, Sue, told me a story about being out to dinner with a friend, Kate, and Kate's father. It was at a fancy restaurant and during the course of an hour and a half Kate's father worked his way through two bottles of wine. Sue was uncomfortable at the idea of Kate's dad driving her home and excused herself from the table. It was in the days before cell phones so she asked the maître d' at the front of the restaurant to use his phone. She called and asked her mom to come get her, telling her she was ill and needed to go home. Mom agreed and came to get her.

Sue told her mom that Kate's father, who had driven them to the restaurant, had been drinking. Her mom offered to drive Kate home, too, but Kate refused. Suffice it to say, it was an uncomfortable moment for everyone. Kate and her father left first. Sue and her mother followed a little while later. As they drove home they passed Kate and her father, who had been pulled over by the highway patrol. So, they ended up taking Kate home anyway while the police escorted her father to jail. Ask yourself, would you or your child have the courage to act the same way that young lady did?

Encouraging discriminating compliance is not intended to invite anarchy into your home. Trusting your gut begins with teaching your gut to listen.

keep your own biases in mind

The challenge lies in helping your child figure out when to go along with an authority figure and when to question authority. To assist a child in making that judgment, adults must examine their own beliefs about authority. Do you blindly accept the word of authority figures? Do you accept that authority figures are not perfect? Do you understand the risk of victimization if children are taught to blindly accept authority? Children very often learn their behavior from their parents. A parent who never trusts a police officer will raise a child to never ask a police officer for help. A parent who never questions a religious or sports figure will raise a child who is likely to do the same. Many of the facts about abuse underscore how important discrimination is. Those who were abused by an authority figure are more likely to be abusive in their own turn. And many victims are raised by parents who not only don't question authority figures, but unwittingly give them their support.

Help your child understand the thought process behind her decisions. Teach your child to think for herself. Encourage your child to say no when things don't feel right, and that it is okay to demand an explanation when something seems off. And, always, encourage your child to communicate their feelings and experiences to people both you and they trust.

twelve

know when NOT to mind your manners

Teach your kids it's okay to:

avoid people they don't know;

say no if they feel uncomfortable;

ask you for permission first; and

trust their gut.

Wait a minute! First you tell me to teach my children to be polite to cops. Then you tell me to teach them to question the authority of teachers and coaches. And now you are saying they shouldn't be polite at all. How does that make sense?

the importance of being impolite

Think about it in terms of safety. It makes perfect sense. Thinking critically, communicating, using knowledge: We've talked about these things again and again. Knowing that a police officer can offer help in a crisis is knowledge. Learning to trust and train your gut as you encounter any authority figure is knowledge and communication. Assessing a situation and what makes safe sense boils down to critical thinking. Anything—unquestioned acceptance of an authority figure, or manners over safety—that undercuts critical thinking can undercut personal safety.

Of course, parents teaching young children how to thrive in the world encourage good manners. We teach our kids to say hello to people they don't know, to shake their hands. We may also urge them to hug, kiss the cheek of, and even to sit on the laps of people we may know well but who are utter strangers to them. We teach them that a thoughtful child should speak when spoken to and always be helpful when asked. These polite and dutiful children are a delight to have around, but they are also a potential target for a would-be abductor. Which is why children need to know that there are times when they can and, in fact, should ignore the rules about being polite.

teaching smart rudeness

Just as we said in the previous chapter: It's okay to say no to Uncle Elmer's lap and, taking it a step further, your child needs to know that it is okay to avoid talking to strangers and that they can turn down a plea for help. This isn't impolite behavior; it is safe behavior.

As I've said elsewhere, children should be taught that if a car pulls over to the side of the road anywhere near them, they should get away quickly. That it may be someone just wanting directions doesn't matter. Step away quickly, ideally cross the street if it is safe to do so. Do not wait until the driver or passenger speaks to you, but act immediately. It has been demonstrated over and over that kids can be told until the cows come home how to act when approached by a stranger, but once in conversation with a stranger they will repeatedly do the opposite. Why? Because we have all been taught to be polite.

The lost puppy or kitten story is often the most difficult for kids to resist. There are many videos that show kids heading off to look for a lost puppy, despite having just been told at length not to help strangers look for lost puppies. Why do they do it? Children live in the moment and are often driven by instant gratification. They have also been told to be helpful, respect their elders, and demonstrate good manners. That, in combination with the idea of finding a puppy, erases the rule to avoid strangers. So keep reminding your children of the rules and know that practice can help. Repeat the lesson. Explain to your child that when someone asks for help, the child should come and get you. If your child is old enough, explain that very often there is no puppy. If your child is younger, explain that the surest way to help find the lost animal is to find you first.

So what to do? Practice, practice, practice.

The more realistic the practice, the better. Send someone your child does not know to drive by and ask for help. Watch to see what happens. Did your child step closer to the car to talk or did she get away from the car when it slowed down? If your daughter did not move quickly to get away from the car, discuss how and why she made her decision with her. Don't frighten her, just teach. Teach your children that there are times when it is necessary to "never mind your manners."

never mind your manners

Two personal experiences helped make the message of "never mind your manners" crystal clear to me. The first occurred when one of the five children in my home was playing in an open field close to the house. I live in a rural area where unwisely, but frequently, people tend to drop their guard and let children play unattended. On this day, I was guilty of that same oversight. One of my children came into the house with a phone number a man had given him. He told me the man was out of gas and had asked him to call his friend to bring some gasoline. Fixated on the fact that my child had not only been approached, but had also gotten close enough to a stranger to walk off with a scribbled phone number, I ran out the door in a panic. I was ready to challenge this man who had approached my child. My son was mortified. Later I would take a good hour to explain my concerns and consequent reaction to my son. What was strange was that when I went out to confront him, neither the man nor the car were to be found. Did he figure he had enough gas to get home? Get spooked? Get bored? Receive help from someone else? What was he after? Of course, I'll never know.

The second experience involved a stranger and a brand-new bicycle. My middle stepson raced into the house one day explaining that a man in an old red truck had just pulled up and asked him to come over. The man had said that he had a brand-new bike in his truck and was about to take it to the dump. With my son standing on the other side of the street, the man had been forced to call out the question "Would you like it?" My stepson thought quickly. He was discerning enough to realize that the man's offer was odd, so he came in the house to talk with me. Heading outside, I saw the truck driving off down the street with the bike in the back. Once again, I really don't know what this stranger was after. As before, he did not stick around so I could ask. Perhaps this man really did want to give away a new bike that was otherwise headed for the dump, though I'm skeptical. Thanks to the fact that my stepson was prepared to risk a free bike to check with me first, I never had to have my skepticism confirmed.

Recently a friend of mine told me an interesting story about her twelve-year-old son. It seemed a "nice lady and man" had befriended him in a local bagel shop. Her son had begun a ritual of walking to the bagel store every Saturday to meet a friend and pick up bagels for the family. The shop was on a busy street in his medium-size town, and she had felt very comfortable that he would be safe walking there. She also liked the idea that her son could practice his independence in a safe environment. He had been going there for about six months without incident.

On one very rainy morning she decided to drive him to the store and to wait outside as he ran in. After about ten minutes she got impatient and went in to see what was taking so long. When she entered the store she saw her son and his friend sitting at a table with a middle-aged couple. The man was showing the boys card tricks and both were watching closely. At first she did not think much of it, but when the boys stood up and said "see you next week," she flashed on a story I had told her months before about a kindly gentleman who my stepson (yes, the same stepson) had met at the mall.

This man had twice bought my fourteen-year-old stepson lunch at McDonald's and had encouraged him to call him anytime he wanted lunch or even to see a movie. My stepson thought he had discovered a free meal plan and enthusiastically shared the news with me. In my usual role as a killjoy, I pointed out to him how odd this seemed since he didn't know this man and I encouraged him to delete the man's number from his phone. After some discussion, he agreed it was indeed a bit odd, and the number was deleted. My stepson reported seeing the man a few times afterward and said each time he had walked by without even acknowledging him. I heartily encouraged my stepson's "rudeness." And I applauded the fact that he had not given his phone number to the man.

Back to the bagel shop: After flashing on what I'd told her, my friend thought she should meet the couple who seemed to know her child so well; she walked over and introduced herself. They shook hands. She asked if they were new to the area and they answered yes. They seemed nice enough, but she had a bad feeling when they could not agree on what their local home address was. Her question had not been intended as a trap; she had been genuinely curious as to where they lived.

On the ride home her son told her that the couple had intro-duced themselves about two months before. They had offered the two boys a hot chocolate after a long conversation regarding baseball and the boys' clothing. The first week the boys had turned them down but by the third week of regularly running into the couple they readily accepted, believing it would have been rude not to, now that they kind of "knew" each other. And they enjoyed talking to the couple about baseball and other topics relevant to twelve-year-olds. Her son's friend reported thinking it was a bit weird that the lady started to ask him to "bring their 'girlfriends' to the shop on Saturdays" when they came, a topic he was not really comfortable with, but by then everyone was familiar with the routine and so for two months these spontaneous conversations continued every Saturday morning. When my friend told her husband what was happening, and that it left her feeling nervous, he thought she was overreacting. After all, they lived in a friendly town and the couple was just being nice. Most people, after all, are nice. The fact that they didn't seem to know their own address? He responded, "New addresses can be confusing." Perhaps their confusion was an honest mistake. The fact that baseball was giving way to inviting girls? Just a shift in topics. Possibly.

The following week Saturday rolled around and the mom suggested that she go into the shop again. The boys objected, saying they were not little kids, but the mom insisted. When they walked in, the couple was not there. In fact, three weeks later they still had not returned. Does this mean that they represented a danger to these two boys? Of course neither my friend nor I know the answer to that. Maybe they went on a diet and stopped eating bagels, or perhaps they really had other ideas for the boys and didn't like answering a mother's questions. But speculating about the couple's motives is the lesser point. The more important point is that the courtesy of the boys opened them up to a potential danger, which only came to light by accident.

understanding the gray area

Many children are raised in strict, what might even be called authoritarian, households. These are homes in which the parents claim final and complete authority and their children are taught to accept and never challenge. This approach to child rearing might be an effective way for busy parents to manage hectic schedules, particularly when their children are young, but it creates its own challenges.

If you teach your child to blindly comply with whatever you say, then how will you teach him that there are times he *should* challenge and go against authority? "What?" you ask. "I want my daughter to do exactly as I say, when I say it." Of course, your child does need to listen to you, and she needs to follow your instructions, but as she grows up she also needs to learn to think for herself and to practice making good choices. The challenge is to teach children to be smart about their safety, which means teaching them to think for themselves. Polite kids, yes; kids who pay attention and do what their parents ask of them, yes. But kids trained to politely do whatever an adult says, no. A parent cannot be in every outdoor field, every mall, every bagel shop; no parent should actually want to. What every parent wants are smart, capable kids who can think for themselves.

If you teach your child that life really does come in shades of gray, you are teaching her how to cope with difficult and confusing situations. If something seems odd—a free bike, special privileges from a teacher or coach, repeat attention from a stranger—she needs to know to question it, and talk to you about it. Not every question has an easy answer; things are not all good or all bad. It is critical that you teach your kids to feel comfortable asking you questions, but it is also critical that they learn to think on their own. Don't wait until your child is sixteen to ask him: "If everyone else jumps off a cliff would you jump too?" The best way to prevent your children from being taken advantage of is to teach them early on the importance of thinking things through. This can begin with teaching that sometimes it is important for kids to "never mind their manners." This opens up the conversation that rules vary depending on different settings, as does trust. Help support the notion that an adult needs to earn a child's trust. For example, teachers should be believed and listened to, but even in a school setting a child's independent judgment should be encouraged. Teach children that it is okay to ask questions, reserve their opinion, and weigh suggestions and requests. And most important, open the lines of communication between you and your children and your children's friends. You want them to ask you questions as you guide them safely into adulthood.

false allegations

If you suspect abuse:
> first, ensure your safety and your child's safety;
>
> review the Safety Equation;
>
> report it to appropriate agencies; and
>
> don't jump to conclusions.

don't jump to conclusions

One of the dangers in writing a book on keeping children safe is it can encourage and even create an environment of paranoia. We are all prone to it. My sister, for example, was convinced she had spied a potential threat at her local gym. She was there at the same time eight local male high school athletes came in for their workout. She then noticed a rather odd-looking guy working out at the same time who kept glancing over at the boys. He also appeared to be posturing for the boys, catching their attention by lifting very heavy weights, and displaying his technique in what looked like a demonstration of his strength. *Aha!* my sister thought, *a creeper right here at my own gym!*

At one point the man went over to one of the boys and asked who had taught him a particular weight-lifting move. The boy answered and the man proceeded to give the boy instructional tips on weight lifting. *Oh, how can he be so bold to do that right in front of me?* my sister thought. *Creep!* She was shocked to find this brazenly happening in her own little town and beginning to wonder just what she ought to do about it.

And then she realized the man was their coach.

Three of the boys approached him, called him coach, and asked him a question about their particular workouts. Everything fell into place. Of course he was checking them out; of course he was monitoring them. It was his job to oversee their workouts, to look at them with frequency, and show them proper technique while also giving them instruction about their workout routines.

This experience really struck a chord with my sister, and makes the point: We have to be careful about leaping to conclusions and convicting people when we don't know the entire story.

Do not misunderstand me. The big takeaway message is, was, and will always remain: If a child has any reason to be concerned for her safety, she should act immediately to ensure it. Cross the street; don't help find the lost puppy; don't accept the ride with the stranger; be rude if you have to. But staying safe is a very different subject than accusing someone of misconduct. That driver may indeed just be lost, the puppy may indeed need to be found, and the stranger may in fact be nothing but well intentioned; and, in each instance, those are facts that can be investigated later. The point is that intuition, experience, and knowledge can help keep you safe; once you are safe, act judiciously before making any accusation.

In one situation I am familiar with, twin boys reported that they had been sexually molested by their grandfather. A full-blown trial followed that raised more questions than answers. Both attorneys appeared fully invested in their clients' viewpoints. The boys' therapist was absolutely sure the boys had been molested based on their behavior. Neighbors, professionals, and some relatives all professed their belief that the grandfather was innocent: the son-in-law (father of the boys) was certain that the grandfather was a sexual predator. "The boys were violated," he declared publicly; he was absolutely certain his wife's father was guilty. Eventually, it came out that an anonymous older woman, someone in her midseventies, had called the local child abuse hotline to report that the twins were being sexually abused. Three additional anonymous calls were made before the authorities stepped in. At first, the boys expressed uncertainty, but in time they began to state that it was true, their grandfather had molested them. In fact, the more they were interviewed, the more sure they became.

Crucial to the case were the statements of the boys' therapist. The therapist reported that at first she had seen no indication of abuse, but after a second interview with police, she acknowledged concerns regarding the boys' behavior. She cited an example of a session that the boys had attended with their grandfather, who had brought them. When she went to the waiting room she found the boys sitting very close to their grandfather. She considered this very unusual behavior for men. She went on to say that, in addition, one of the boys had gained a tremendous amount of weight during the year. She declared that weight gain was an indicator of sexual abuse.

Except there is no clinical evidence that shows weight gain corresponds to sexual abuse, and fathers and grandfathers sit close to their children and grandchildren all the time. So did the therapist mean to mislead the police? It *does* make sense that kids might gain weight if they are abused. It *does* make sense that a predator might keep children especially close to him. But drawing those connections begins with the assumption that the accusation has merit; neither fact on its own is in any way conclusive.

In the case of the twin boys, things got really out of hand. The parents separated during the trial, at the end of which a jury found the evidence insufficient to reach a guilty verdict. This did not keep the grandfather from being treated with doubt and suspicion by family and friends. This meant that the family did not ever want him to be alone with his grandchildren or for that matter any other child again. Although he was not placed on California's Megan's list for convicted sex offenders, he was known to the local authorities as having a *possible* sexual violation. They would respond just a little quicker if another allegation popped up. The consequence for this grandfather was the loss of his family.

In divorce cases allegations are often used as a weapon between parents. Once an accusation is introduced everyone becomes a little more careful. The questions loom large: What if it happened? What if it didn't? Judges, therapists, families, and attorneys have a very difficult time sorting it all out. I have worked with numerous patients in high-conflict divorces. Sometimes it is clearly established that a parent did indeed molest a child. Sometimes, however, it is not at all clear what took place.

the line between safety and accusation

Safety and accusation are not the same. Do you have concerns about a coach, teacher, or anyone else? Talk to your child. Take steps to prevent her from being alone with that person. A suspicion is more than enough to justify a parent taking steps to protect a child. However, suspicion isn't enough to level an accusation. But it sure should encourage a concerned caregiver to learn more facts and discover what's up. Again, educate your child on the safety protocols covered in this book—make sure a parent or caregiver always knows where they are, with whom, how they can be reached, and where they will be. Teach kids to be alert and to think things through. The big messages of the book remain no less true: Communication is king, and education is power. And only from a position of open communication and knowledge of the facts should someone take legal steps to bring concerns to proper authorities. Once you are confident that you've looked to your child's safety, consider what you know and what you don't, who you can and should talk to, and what the next steps are depending on what you learn. Act quickly to ensure your children are safe; act deliberately and thoughtfully and through proper legal channels when leveling an accusation of improper behavior.

Resources for Reporting Improper Behavior

- Contact the police.
- Contact Child Protective Services.
- Childhelp USA National Child Abuse Hotline: 1-800-422-4453.

coaches: a case study

Coaches are all over the news. A few bad ones have been receiving extensive attention for the despicable acts they have committed against kids. At the same time, and often in the very same newspapers and on TV news shows, the fabulous athletic achievements of hardworking kids and their schools are being celebrated. No one denies that for the most part coaches are unsung heroes; many work for little or no pay and are instrumental in helping to form the character of countless kids. If these men and women are doing their jobs correctly, they are working closely with children, forging relationships that can be very intimate. Athletic performance is necessarily part physical and part emotional, because if you're to compete, motivation, stress, and the fear of failure and success are always with you. That kind of intense intimacy can create skilled athletes, local, even state champs, sometimes Olympic stars. It can also, on rare occasions, create an opportunity for abuse.

Many coaches enter our children's lives when the kids are in middle school and high school, or precisely when they are beginning the process of separating from their parents and when they are particularly susceptible to the influence of other adults. When your children enter the age range of middle through high school, you need to talk with them about appropriate relationships with adults, including the necessity of maintaining healthy boundaries. A child is far more likely to let a parent know what is going on if, first, she has been told what appropriate and inappropriate behavior is for an adult and, second, she knows that if something comes up that makes her uncomfortable she can tell her parent and not be blamed. Again, communication is king.

Dealing with Blurred Boundaries

What would you do in these difficult situations?

- A coach wants to take your fifteen-year-old daughter to a concert to see her favorite band, alone. He says it's her reward for being his best player.

    Suggest that if he'd like to give her tickets as a reward, you would be happy to take her, but you don't think it's appropriate for him to take her alone.

- Your six-year-old tells you that she doesn't like it when Uncle Tim makes her sit on his lap. He likes to tickle her and even though she likes him, she hates it when he does this. She begs you not to say anything.

    Tell her that you're glad she said something. And remind your daughter that it's okay to say no next time Uncle Tim asks her. Let your daughter know that you will stay nearby when Uncle Tim is around and make sure you are there to supervise the visit. Let her know that you will tell Uncle Tim that you are happy he is there, but do not want your daughter to sit on his lap when he is visiting. Remind her that this is a good way to learn to stick up for herself and that she has not done or said anything wrong!

- At your son's school you are the one who volunteers for all the classroom activities. Well, you don't exactly volunteer, other parents seem to sign you up; they always say, "We knew you wouldn't mind." Well, you do mind. It's beginning to interfere with your life at home and you don't have time to help your own children. Your son thinks it's great that you do so much.

Tell your son that you love him and you like helping out but you need to draw some boundaries. From now on, only make yourself available for the things you have time to do and let the other parents know that you are making a change and are not available except when you sign yourself up.

A safety equation can be a great help with this age group. So we start with a female high school softball player and a coach who thinks she's very talented. So far, so good. The girl is shaping up to be the real star of the team and the coach is spending extra time working with her, perfecting her skills. So far this just means more time spent after school on the softball field. Okay, good athlete + interested coach + public practice area = safe situation.

Let's assume her mom believes her daughter deserves the extra attention; after all, the word is that her daughter can earn a college scholarship, maybe even make it to the Olympics. She's heard from the coach and friends that her daughter is special. The daughter feels the same way, and is so dedicated that she even has a ringtone on her phone just so her coach can reach her day or night. Coach suggests they do a little more one-on-one work. Maybe some hydrotherapy at the pool to strengthen her quads. He has a pool at his house so they won't be interrupted. By the way, this coach is new to the high school and no one knows much about him. He *seems* okay; the school wouldn't hire someone dangerous, would they? Besides, the daughter is *really* talented, and a scholarship would make all the difference. Uh-oh, this is getting a little more complicated. But not from the vantage point of the safety equation. Just adding in "new coach" shifts the outcome just enough to raise a question. Let's change the equation even more: After the one-on-one hydrotherapy session the girl seems to lose interest in playing softball, cancels that ringtone, starts to practice less. Interested new coach + private time + suddenly disinterested talented athlete = What's going on here? = potential risk.

If alarm bells aren't ringing yet, they should be. Now the team is traveling for play-offs. The coach is concerned about the health of his star player, even suggests that she sleep in his hotel room to ensure "she gets a good night's sleep." Coach also implies that Mom needs to let go a little if she wants her daughter to be successful. The daughter says she doesn't want to talk about it. Now those alarm bells are really starting to ring. And when those bells start sounding, it's time to start gathering information, opening up lines of communication.

What if the coach is well known with an unblemished record and numerous testimonials to his skill and dedication to his players? What if the coach is a woman? What if Mom hears from one of her daughter's friends that her daughter is being bullied by a jealous teammate and the coach is protecting her? What if the daughter swears up and down that there is nothing inappropriate going on? When should Mom take further steps, and when should she urge others with proper authority to look into things?

Interested coach spending more and more unsupervised time with talented, just-turned fifteen-year-old athlete who has suddenly begun to lose interest in the sport = danger. Very-well-known coach with no history of inappropriate behavior, protecting star athlete from bullying = ?? The equation changes with each new piece of information.

This situation comes from a true story told to me by a client. Fortunately, my client did not have to go through criminal proceedings and a trial. She told her mom when and where the coach wanted to meet her alone. She told her mother that something didn't feel right about the relationship. Her mom became suspicious and pressed the school to look into the coach's behavior. She did not make an accusation, she just asked for more information. In this case, it was discovered that the coach had a prior conviction for statutory rape of a fourteen-year-old in another state. My client was not a victim because she and her mother were alert. The mom took action to keep her daughter safe. When the truth came tumbling out many people were shocked. My client went on to have a stellar softball career at an excellent college and is now coaching softball herself.

So what is the right thing to do? What's an overreaction, and what's being too permissive? Suspicion should encourage a concerned parent to learn more facts and discover what's up. Suspicion is more than enough to get an alert child to protect herself. Again, communicate with your child. Again, educate your child on the safety protocols covered in this book. The safety equation always feels different when a parent knows where his kids are, with whom, and how they can be reached. Teach kids to be alert, to think things through, and to tell someone when something doesn't feel right. The case study of coaches captures the bigger point: First ensure a child's safety, and then learn all the facts. Suspicion isn't enough to level an accusation, but it is enough to get you to act to make sure a child is safe.

fourteen

love equals strength

The key to keeping your children safe is to remember:
communication is key;
education is power; and
love is strength.

the power of love

You likely already know that your children learn from you all the time, picking up words, gestures, and ideas. Many kids also walk around with tangible tokens of your affection—things you have bought for them, from jewelry to that pair of must-have sneakers. What you may not know is that these lessons and objects shape their behavior and their ability to stand up for themselves. Why? Because few things help a child more than being confident of your unconditional love.

In the worst of circumstances, love is a source of strength. I know that survivors frequently lean on faith to pull them through adversity. Even nonbelievers lean on something intangible to keep them going. A client of mine, whose daughter had been abducted, wished that she could have given something to her child that symbolized her unending love and the promise of eventual rescue. She wished she could have somehow conveyed the promise to her that she would always be there for her no matter what.

Don't wait to convey the same message to your children. The

thing is that your children take that information with them wherever they go, every day, as long as you keep giving them that message. I worked with a woman who regretted deeply not telling her daughter how she felt, or giving her a tangible sign of her love, something they could both cling to if something bad happened. Something bad did happen. The father took the child out of the country, violating the custody agreement. My client was racked by guilt. There was no way she could send a message of love to her abducted child. "My daughter is all alone, and has nothing from me that could comfort her," she would say to me. But when her daughter was returned to her, she learned that her daughter had held on to a particular memory of the two of them preparing a special meal together. "Mom, I played the scene over and over in my mind when I felt sad, and I felt so close to you." The mother had powerfully conveyed her unconditional love through her actions, allowing the girl to confidently say, "I knew you were there waiting for me."

reinforcing love

The love you give your child turns into the love that they learn to give themselves. Later, when they find themselves in stressful or difficult situations, they are able to call upon that love. We often assume that our children know that we love them unconditionally. We assume they understand that we don't love them just because they score the winning touchdown, or get a ninety-seven on a math test. We love them no matter what happens, even during those times when they irritate and frustrate us. Don't assume. Kids need constant reinforcement. They do worry about not being good enough; they do worry about making choices that will disappoint you. It is a tragic truth that some sexually exploited girls are manipulated by their abusers with threats that shameful photographs will be shown to their parents if they don't do what is asked or demanded of them. Perversely, this frequently keeps the teen from breaking away because they are afraid that the parents "cannot possibly love me after that!" What if that child knows in her heart that she will be understood and loved unconditionally?

Parental disapproval is a double-edged sword. Fear of it can often work in a positive way. It can be the voice of conscience that keeps kids out of trouble. But it can also prevent kids from trusting themselves. Not trusting yourself keeps you from advocating for yourself. And not trusting yourself can lead you to think: *It doesn't matter what I do anyway. Nobody cares.* So tell your children that you love them! Tell them what they mean to you and let them know that you will always be there for them. If you treat them with love and respect, they will love and respect themselves. It will help them through the tough times, and it will help you, too.

What's the downside? There isn't any. Telling a child or a teen over and over again that you love them and will be there for them regardless is at worst a slight embarrassment to your child (though that is likely more show than real). It doesn't mean that they are excused to do whatever they want. Letting your child get away with bad behavior is no substitute to showing them unconditional love. The latter has nothing to do with how and where you set limits. Children who never have boundaries set for them are notoriously bad at setting boundaries for themselves. But knowing how much you love him or her gives your child a clear and absolute power in the world. Against all of life's challenges, your love is a powerful antidote.

How do we do this in practical terms? Our love is expressed through our words and deeds. As parents, most of us do both without thinking. Learning to think about it and making a more conscious effort to express your love will be noticed by your child. Sometimes, personal circumstances make this hard. A bad divorce or, for whatever reason, an unhappy household can strain words and deeds. But making clear how much you love your children is probably the easiest thing you can do, far easier than paying for a grand vacation or resolving a tense relationship between spouses or exes. Indeed, when both parents make expressing love for their kids a priority, alongside safety, it can improve tense and difficult relationships and divorces. If circumstances are difficult, your children will probably be less giving in return. Don't let that stop you. Nothing will get across your unconditional love than to extend it without condition. Remember, they are looking to you. Your strength is theirs. And be confident that no matter what they reflect back to you, showing them your absolute love will make them stronger, and it will keep them safer.

Simple Ways to Show Your Love

- Tell them you love them.
- Hug and kiss your children, especially when they are leaving or coming home.
- Leave notes for them.
- Spend time together: Playing and cooking together are two great activities!
- Listen attentively when they talk to you. Stop what you are doing and focus.
- Eat dinner together as much as possible.
- Display their creative work.
- Encourage your children's dreams.

fifteen

flexibility and the survivor gene

Train your children to be survivors:

    Shake up routines and schedules.

    Teach adaptability.

    Show them frustration is manageable.

    Teach coping strategies.

What is the scariest situation you can imagine? When asked, one of my clients declared unhesitatingly that being on a plane for even a moment would terrify her. She told me she had never flown and whenever she even tried to convince herself to take a trip, she just could not muster up enough courage. Many of us are afraid to fly, but we learn to manage those fears, maybe out of necessity or to enjoy the rewards that come with air travel. This client had lived her life so that she need never step on a plane, and she was confident that she would never need to. She was unwilling to develop the skills necessary to manage her fear of flying. Without question, her life was consequently limited. The people, sights, and experiences available to us by flying to distant cities and countries will forever remain beyond her easy grasp. Unable to accept change, unwilling to learn how to conquer fear and adapt, she will spend most of her life in one small area.

What allows one person to overcome a fear of flying, but leaves another person hopelessly trapped by the same fear? It is very tempting to look for absolute truths about human nature, to believe we can find a clear and unambiguous answer to who is capable of overcoming adversity and surviving calamity. But perceiving the world as black and white can blind us to a simple truth: There are no absolutes, each of us is different, and there is no one "right" way. Personality differences, lessons learned in childhood (whether positive or negative), coping strategies, and the ability to tolerate and accept distress are all factors in managing and overcoming our fears.

the survivor gene

In his book *The Survivors Club: The Secrets and Science That Could Save Your Life*, Ben Sherwood highlights the stories of a handful of survivors and discovers that they had many traits in common, particularly optimism and a sense of spirituality. Based on some convincing research, Sherwood suggests that there may be such a thing as a survival gene. We might inherit our ability to survive, and it may be more evolved in some than in others. But what if that is only part of the picture? Perhaps resiliency varies from situation to situation as much as if not more so than from person to person. Maybe the ability to survive depends on one's frame of mind at the time of crisis. Certainly, all of the survivors in Sherwood's book agree that a positive outlook was crucial to their survival.

stay calm

For many lucky people getting on an airplane doesn't cause a second of distress. For others, it's an awful experience and trying to get over it is more difficult than just not getting on the plane in the first place. Most of us live between these two extremes: We can easily manage a twinge of anxiety at the door of the airplane or we can learn to adapt to the circumstances. The majority of us won't ever be in a situation where we have to test our survival gene, but all of us will experience stress and anxiety in some form, regardless of our age. We all know that how we cope with stressful situations can contribute greatly to our overall health. Learning how to stay calm, grounded, and centered, and utilizing well-developed coping strategies are crucial to taking care of yourself and those around you. Many people don't have any coping strategies at all; you will give your children a great gift if you can help them develop some of their own.

More and more clinicians have found evidence that positive thought processes help with some types of depression. Optimism is a positive coping skill and should be supported and even fostered in children as they develop. So how does all this line up with a book about being wise and teaching our children to avoid harmful situations? Here's how: The ability to remain calm is a learned skill, and it is a skill that directly contributes to safety. We can help our children by teaching them to stay calm and centered in adverse situations. We can teach them to put both feet on the ground, breathe, and stay focused on the present moment. Some schools in California provide earthquake kits to the younger school-age children. Parents are asked to provide a letter reminding their child to "stay calm, you are loved, and someone will be there as soon as possible." The purpose is obvious. With each of my children, I remember thinking how uncomfortable it was to write this letter, but also how reassuring it was to think they would have that note if anything happened.

Teaching a child how to remain calm is really hard, especially if you are the type of parent who tends to overreact. Having an accurate sense of yourself is important, so briefly think about it. How have you reacted in situations of stress or crisis? What lessons do you think your child has learned as she watched your reactions? One friend told us she grew up in a house where everyone overreacted; everything was a big drama. She told us it was not until she began riding horses that she learned just how much she, too, overreacted to every situation, large or small. Because their very survival depends on their ability to assess potential danger, horses have a natural ability to pick up on our stress levels, which in turn provides a constant feedback loop to the attentive rider. Our friend used her experience with horses to teach herself how to stay calm when frightened. If she overreacted when she was around the horses, they would inevitably respond by overreacting too, shying away from jumps, trying to buck or rear, and acting in ways that showed they were supersensitive to her reactions. In time she passed what she had learned from the horses on to her two children. And now they all practice breathing slowly when stressed out and sitting quietly for a few minutes each morning.

Calming Skills to Practice with Your Children

- Focus on what is in the here and now, instead of the past or future.
- Stay in the present moment. Count four or five things that you can see around you. Now count four or five things you can feel. Now count four or five things you can hear.
- Practice feeling the place where your breath goes in and out.
- Put both of your feet on the floor, slow your breathing down, and practice letting go of the tension from the top of your head to the tip of your toes. Feel the support of the chair underneath you.
- Count to five while you inhale. Count to five while you exhale. Relax your shoulders.

It doesn't require reams of scientific data to conclude that learning to remain calm is better than giving in to anxiety, that self-confidence is preferable to fear, and hopefulness more helpful than depression. And my practical experience and understanding of the emerging literature point me toward one more insight, the importance of flexibility.

Along with optimism, all of the survivors Sherwood chronicled in *The Survivors Club* had mastered flexibility to one degree or another.

be flexible

What does *flexibility* mean in practical terms? *Flexibility* means the ability to adjust to changing circumstances. In order to negotiate the world, we develop patterns of thinking, assumptions, and beliefs that allow us to make quick judgments, and to react appropriately to situations. It is easy, particularly as we get older, to become rigid thinkers, to get stuck in patterns. Imagine your daughter comes home reporting she doesn't like the way her teacher gives directions. How do you respond? What lessons will your response impart? Do you try immediately to get the school to put your daughter in a different class, or might you help your child more if, while you gain more information, you explain to her that people do things in different ways? By teaching her flexibility, the skill of adjusting and adapting, you prepare her for the inevitable moment when you won't be there to buffer her from someone's negative behavior. Examine your willingness as a parent to allow your child to maneuver through life's challenges and so develop her flexibility. Look for chances to support your child's coping skills.

For one friend, that opportunity arose when her young child witnessed his school administrator give a trespassing teenager a bloody nose when he jerked a book out of the older student's hands. The teenager shouldn't have been trespassing, yes. The administrator overreacted, yes. The altercation between the two was upsetting for my friend's young child, as well as the four or five other children who witnessed it. Weeks later, the administrator released his own version of the story. In fact, he announced that the children who had witnessed the event had lied when describing it. He flatly declared that what they reported had never happened.

The young children who had observed the altercation were crushed by the discrepancy between what they had seen and what the administrator now claimed. Adults in the community were polarized, with many believing the children were lying, and others demanding that the administrator resign. My friend discussed the events with her son throughout the year. She also weighed the merits of keeping the child in the school versus moving him to a new school. As these things often go, it was more than a year before the administrator left and the story was never completely substantiated either way. Even now, eleven years later, people have different opinions about what happened.

But good did arise from an otherwise bad situation. Yes, my friend's son was exposed to the sad reality that people don't always take children at their word, but he also learned that he had the ability to remain flexible as this administrator stayed on for another year and a half. The whole incident was an unfortunate experience for an impressionable child, but was made the better by his mother's ability to seize the opportunity to discuss with him the complexities of the issue, to encourage his coping strategies, and to help him learn to adapt.

The ability to survive may be a trait we are born with, but much like a shyness gene, it does not a personality make. We used to believe a shy child should be supported in their shyness because, after all, "that is who they are." Now we teach children to leave their comfort zone and try something different. The ability to survive may indeed come from an inborn gene, but we can teach children to stretch, and in so doing become stronger. Norman Doidge challenges the notion of a hardwired, unchanging brain in his book *The Brain That Changes Itself*. In it he argues that breakthroughs in neuroscience show how, through thought and activity, the brain exhibits the ability to change its own structure. It literally adapts to circumstances.

how do you respond to challenges?

An important tip with all children is to limit the lecture and model the behavior. So before you ask how adaptable your children are, ask yourself how easily you adapt to changes. Do you resist new technologies, or do you embrace them, pushing yourself to learn how to use them? Are you listening to the same music you listened to as a teen, or are you exploring new and different artists? As we get older it is harder and harder to be flexible. That is all the more reason to push yourself to develop flexibility in order to respond to change. Talk to your child early on about your own difficulties coping with change, using that admission as a way of challenging both of you to overcome a reluctance to embrace flexibility. Ask yourself, do I positively model flexibility/adjustment/adaptation? Positive adaptation might include expressing disappointment when something goes a little differently than expected, but showing your child how you still managed to adjust. Keep in mind that children learn by doing, but also by watching what the adults around them do. Don't burden them with your own internal process, but allow them to see how you or other significant caregivers tackle challenges.

Do you ask your children about how they are managing the stress in their lives? Maybe you could talk about this after a particularly difficult test at school, or when they have been confronted with a tense situation. "How did that make you feel?" "What did you do to manage that?" "Were you afraid?" Let your curiosity guide you and really listen to their responses. You might learn something useful, too!

Attitude may not be everything, but it certainly can help promote awareness and a willingness to carry on. Again, flexibility is the ability to adapt to a situation without letting it crush you, and having that ability can make all the difference in surviving and eventually recovering from abduction or other traumatic experiences.

sixteen

when do we tell the kids?

When talking to kids, remember two things:
> their developmental age (level of maturity) and
> to ask questions.

Each child is different. Kids might all have similar patterns of growing, but they all grow at different speeds. I know, I know, you have heard that a hundred times, but it's true. These differences have a lot to do with when and how you talk to children about difficult topics. There is a set of twins I know, let's call them Anne and Michelle, who have always done everything differently, even though they were born only five minutes apart. When they were babies, Anne was bigger than Michelle and walked months before her sister. By the time they were both preteens, Michelle eventually grew to be six inches taller than her twin. She was more coordinated than Anne and loved to play Little League softball and volleyball at her elementary school. By high school, Michelle stayed about two inches taller, but became quite shy, while Anne became a champion gymnast, had lots of friends, and loved to go to school dances. Everything that was predicted when they were babies changed when they were in elementary school, and changed again when they were in high school. By the time they were teens, the taller one was frightened easily by anything unknown while the shorter one would jump into things feet first.

Sometimes, however, people treat Anne like she is a lot younger than she is just because she is shorter, while the taller Michelle gets treated like she is older and more mature. Looks can be deceiving. For example, while Anne likes to babysit and Michelle gets easily overwhelmed when put in charge of younger children, neighborhood parents often expect Michelle to show up and are concerned when Anne does. On one occasion a parent called their mother to ask for Michelle, worried that when Anne arrived she was not old enough or mature enough to handle the job. Their mom had to reassure the other mother that both girls were the same age and that Anne was fully capable of the job.

Just because a child looks a certain way does not have anything to do with how mature he or she is. Think about the kids you know. Just because they are in a certain grade does not mean they are the same emotional age as their classmates. Emotional age sounds like a big, fancy term but it really is not. It basically means: How well can someone handle difficult topics without getting overwhelmed? Not a very technical definition, but it works for what I mean!

What follows are suggestions as to how parents can introduce tough subjects related to safety for different ages. Keep in mind that emotional age matters, too. Some five-year-olds can handle more complicated safety protocols, and some teens can become paralyzed by details. This is organized by age, but use your best judgment; no one knows your kids better than you do. Some nine-year-olds really are more like six- or eleven-year-olds and we all know grown-ups who act younger than their own children!

ages 2–6: little ones

So you have a two-year-old in your house? These guys are not the best at long conversations. That goes without saying—just note the glazed look you get when you go on for too long. More likely, they will simply get up and start playing or suddenly get really whiny. Too long is often anything over a minute. They do not follow logic easily and are not very good at communicating clearly. They are just beginning to make sentences and often confuse one word for another. They're likely to look at you like you are an alien when you talk to them about concepts and facts they do not understand. Still, they are learning new things every day and for most children this age their language is growing by leaps and bounds. Their storytelling ability can be limited, but don't forget to really listen to them. The story your child tells may be confused, with the ending told at the beginning, but that does not mean the whole story is wrong. One little girl I know was trying to describe a man parked on her street who frightened her. She kept reporting "that man drove away," leaving out the fact that he had been sitting in his car outside their house. Her mom had to listen carefully before she could figure out the child was talking about a real situation and not a pretend story. Then the little girl added something about "the horse on the car," which confused her mother. At first this sounded like a fantasy story. Only later, and because she listened, did she figure out that the man had been in a car with the image of a horse on its trunk—a Ford Mustang. It took some work, but Mom got enough information to make sense out of the story. And because she did, she had the knowledge she needed to be alert, and what to be alert for.

keep it simple

How would you talk about something complicated or scary to kids this age? Obviously, you need to keep it super simple. In fact, most things worth saying to any child regardless of their age are best kept simple. You don't need to use fear to get across the simple rule that Mommy and Daddy or other caregivers need to know where they are at all times. It is easier to tell kids as young as two to six that they must stay close to the person who is taking care of them than to explain all the reasons why. That's the rule, period. Some may be mature enough at that age to sift through the reasons behind the request, but at this age, keep it simple and use your energy to make sure they follow the rules instead of spending time explaining your logic. What is true for all kids, however, is they need practice to get good safety protocols right.

Safety Ground Rules for 2–6-Year-Olds

1. Mom and Dad love you very much and we want to keep you safe and happy. You must NEVER go off anywhere by yourself. Until you get bigger one of us must always come with you wherever you go. We will keep an eye on you.

2. Do not run off ahead when we are out walking. You must keep an eye on me.

3. When I say STOP, you must stop. If you can't do that, you will have to hold my hand. (Follow through on this!)

4. If someone is touching you, tickling you, or hurting you and you don't like it you MUST tell us. No one will be mad at you. It's okay to say no.

Practice can be as simple as taking a child to the store, holding their hand, and reminding them to stay close. Two-to-six-year-olds generally will need lots and lots of reminders about staying close and not wandering away. Some kids are better at this than others. In the old days, we used to see kids wearing leashes to keep them close; a really silly-looking contraption, but when you think about it, it doesn't seem so ridiculous. Which makes more sense? A silly leash or your panic when you rush down store aisles looking for your child? Keeping a hand on a stroller or shopping cart is a good idea—to make sure they understand your message. My husband used to try to scare our kids so they would stay close to him in public places, telling them that the bad guys would get them if they didn't. Eventually, I gave him better words to use, and better practices to follow. Words like "Stay close to me while we are here," and practices like "Let's play until we leave, can you always see where I am?" or "Practice being my shadow—can you follow right behind me for the next seven minutes? I'll time you." (I have found that children like the concept of being timed.) Simple consequences *do* work with kids. Games are an option with young kids, but they do need to learn to behave so remind them that if they run off, they will have to hold your hand (or jacket, or stroller handle if appropriate), but you must follow through and actually do it!! Bribery and threats may work in the moment, but in the long run they will encourage your child to repeat the behavior next time. Sometimes expectations are the simplest and most effective: Telling your child exactly how you expect them to behave, and being certain that they can and will do so, can be a remarkable tool to improve behavior. If you believe your children are capable of good behavior, and expect them to behave well, they often *will* behave well!

Kids this age and a little older may act as if they really get it, but they don't. Or they may get it the moment they're told, but forget it just moments later. By now we are all familiar with the many examples of kids responding eagerly to a fake invitation to help a stranger look for a puppy despite long conversations with their mother or father to never go off with a stranger. Keep practicing, keep reminding them, but remember that the best solution is to keep the younger children within eyesight when out of the house. There is simply no safer way.

Signs of Stress in Very Young Children

All children respond to stress differently, but even very young children can be affected by the moods and emotions of the people around them. Some behaviors to look out for include:

- clinginess or increased crying;
- fear of things that did not scare them before;

- more tantrums or anger;
- difficulty falling or staying asleep;
- change in eating habits;
- acting out trauma in games;
- being less responsive or showing less emotion.

ages 6–9

*Be honest. Really talk to your kids and ask questions
so you know they understand.*

Having kids six to nine years old in your house can be a little bit like living with a police force—a very self-absorbed police force. It is all about them. They like the facts and they want the facts clear. Yes, once again children can differ tremendously in temperament, character, and maturity, but with this age group it is best to keep facts precise and the things they need to understand exact. When you say, "Easy come, easy go" they will want to know what is coming and where it is going. Their brains have only grown enough to begin to understand jokes and rhymes with double meanings. However, they may be able to have longer conversations. One-minute conversations can be expanded to five minutes, but don't expect them to recall everything you've said. To them the skill of having conversations may be just beginning. I have a lovely memory of my son and his cousin at this age, sitting in their booster seats, chatting on and on, with no particular purpose and no beginning, middle, or end.

If you are really lucky, at this age your child might even understand your point of view a little more and may actually let you know they get it. Explaining to them that two Popsicles before dinner are not a good idea because "they will fill you up and you won't want to eat dinner" might actually work. Some kids won't tell you that they understand, but if they stop arguing about it, it just might have made sense to them. If you tell your child that it's safer to stay away from the grown-up who hangs out at the playground but doesn't have any kids, it might make sense to them. The best way to make sure, however, remains practice and supervision.

Safety Ground Rules for 6–9-Year-Olds

Make this list of rules together with your child.

1. Let's make a list of people we trust; the people who care about you. We will keep their phone numbers where you can get them. That way you can call them when you want to. These are the ONLY people who are allowed to pick you up in their car.

2. Be sure never to go anywhere, help anyone, take anything someone gives you, or get in a car without telling us or the person who is taking care of you first. Even if you think we might get mad—let them know!

3. Don't ever go alone. Take a friend when you go someplace.

4. Say no if someone does something to you that you don't like, or makes you uncomfortable. It's okay to say no to people; you aren't being mean, you are standing up for yourself!

5. Tell SOMEONE on your list if something bad happens. They won't get mad at you, and they will help you to figure it out.

6. Don't always believe what people tell you—check it out with someone on your list. Like if someone tells you that you are "supposed" to go somewhere with them and you don't know about this, call someone on your list and ask!

When my children were five and nine something happened that is a great example of how two ages see things differently: It began on a Halloween day in our old neighborhood. At about four in the afternoon the police SWAT team surrounded a neighbor's house, guns drawn. Nothing like it had ever happened before. We lived in a small Northern California town and frankly did not even know that a SWAT team existed in the area. As it happened, my five-year-old daughter had been invited to trick or treat with the little girl who lived in the very house now surrounded by police. Watching it all unfold, she assumed it was a part of Halloween and wanted to go over to her friend's house immediately. When I said no, she cried that I was "ruining the surprise her friend had set up." It was Halloween, after all, and to her the guys on the SWAT team looked like people in costume. On the other hand, my nine-year-old wanted to go help the police, as he believed he had seen someone "smoking" outside the house and was interested in catching the person. Suffice it to say, we all stayed inside and only later in the week discovered that it had been a raid for marijuana sales.

Talking with each child later was a challenge, because each needed something different from me, but they both needed the facts. The five-year-old needed to know she could not go play at her friend's house because we were not sure if it was really safe. We told her that the police had been there because they thought the people living there might be doing something that was against the law; we didn't know if anyone had in fact been arrested, and if so for what, but we didn't want her in the middle of it. The nine-year-old needed the facts so he would not have nightmares about the "bad" neighbors. We told him that the police were there because they thought the people living there might be doing something against the law. We also promised to let him know what had happened as soon as we found out. This is an example of talking with children about the same issue with a different focus depending on their developmental age.

When reading the following, please keep in mind that different children who are the same age might understand differently and thus need different explanations.

ages 9–12

Support their ability to understand how others might feel about
something and look for opportunities to build their confidence.

Okay, so your kids are separating from you a little. They are starting
to practice independence and you just don't seem to be as important
to them in the same way as you used to be. They are more independent and need you to take care of them a little less. Joining clubs,
having the right gadgets and toys, being part of the right group are
really important to kids this age. Boys and girls begin to act a little
differently now; boys may be less willing to talk about personal subjects like body functions than girls. This hesitancy can be important
when talking with kids in this age group about the complex topics
of exploitation and sexual abuse. The boys, already reticent to talk
about sex, can feel doubly shamed if someone is asking them to do
something that makes them uncomfortable. Encourage your child to
express their thoughts and ask questions about all subjects. Remember, no matter how sophisticated they may look and sound, they are
still children and have not fully developed the tools to manage the
adult world. Give them pretend examples of events to help them feel
okay about things that may be happening to them. One mother used
an example of a made-up boy whose camp counselor was exposing
him to porn. Ironically, her child acknowledged that the same was
happening to him with another member of the community. The
example she gave had provided him with a way to talk about a very
difficult topic. No, we are not advocating making things up so you
can talk to your children, just that you look for opportunities to have
discussions about these difficult subjects. These children still need
strong rules to keep them safe and follow through when they break
those rules. Though you should not be getting into arguments about
your reasons why, you should give your reasons so children can continue the process of understanding how to keep themselves safe.

Safety Ground Rules for 9–12-Year-Olds

Notice that with nine-to-twelve-year-olds the language you use can be more inclusive. They are old enough to be part of the discussion, but not to set their own rules.

- Let's make a list of people you and I trust; the people who care about you who you and I know really well. We will keep their phone numbers where you can get them if you need to call someone. These are the ONLY people who are allowed to pick you up in an emergency. Is there anyone else you think should be on this list?

- I believe you are beginning to develop good judgment, but you still need to live by the rules:

  - Never go anywhere, help someone you don't know, take anything from someone you don't know, or get in a car without telling us or the person who is taking care of you first. Even if you think we might get mad, let us know!! We can talk about it, but you must agree to this rule. If you are not able to follow it, I am ready to give you consequences—it's that important!

  - Don't ever go alone. Take a friend when you go someplace. This is very important to your safety!

  - Say no if someone does something to you that you don't like or makes you uncomfortable. You are really learning how to stand up for yourself and how to ask for what you need. You must remember that you can always say no.

  - Tell SOMEONE on your list if something bad happens. We love you and we are here to keep you safe; you need to let us know.

  - Don't always believe what people tell you—check it out with someone on your list. If someone tells you that you are "supposed" to go somewhere with them

and you don't know about this, call someone on your
list and ask! This is basic safety!

ages 12–15

*Let your children know that their opinions are really important by
letting them steer the conversation.*

Okay, so kids at this age can still "hear" you before they focus on becoming more independent again. It's not so easy to pull one over on
this age group, but they are still naïve to the ways of the world and
can be trusting when they should be cautious. They sort of get it, if
they really want to get it. At this age they can carry on lengthy conversations and ask important questions, provided they really want to
take the time to have the conversation with you. Don't be surprised
if you hear that your kid talks forever at their best friend's house, but
only a little bit with you. Parents often say, "She doesn't ever tell me
what's going on. I hear about it from one of her friends!" Boys can
be more factual, accurate, and direct in conversation, while girls tend
to be more tactful as they become more aware of the world around
them. And girls tend to worry more about "taking care" of other people, their feelings in particular. Both genders care a lot about being
just like everyone else at this age; many work to avoid standing out in
any way. Even as they struggle to fit in, however, your preteen is eager
to believe she has value in the world. Support this, because when they
value themselves it becomes second nature for them to make good,
healthy choices. You have to be right behind them, encouraging and
supporting them to make good choices. This is a good time to explain your thoughts behind making rules and engage in discussion.
They still have to follow your rules, but engaging in discussion makes
sense now because it allows them to express their views and shows
them how you think through safety-related situations. Challenge

them when they don't make good choices, and follow through with consequences, but first be sure you have educated them on how and why wise decisions are made. If your child believes that the world is basically a safe place, but that there are a few bad people in it, they might use their awareness and their critical-thinking skills to make smart choices. They are practicing and struggling to find out who they want to be and even why they might want to be that way; they are practicing skills to manage the world around them.

Talking with 13–15-Year-Olds About Safety Ground Rules

This conversation will be even more discussion-oriented. You can encourage independence and still keep an eye on the rules.

- Who are the people who care about you who you and I know really well? Do you have their phone numbers? Do you know that you can call them if you need to? These are the ONLY people who would come pick you up if there was an emergency.

- You are becoming more and more independent, so I want to support you and give you tools. In order to stay safe, you need to agree to these rules:

- Never go anywhere, help anyone you don't know, take anything that someone gives you, or get in a car without telling us or the person who is taking care of you first. We can discuss it, but you must agree to this rule. Why do you think I am telling you this?

  - Don't ever go alone. Take a friend when you go someplace. This is very important to your safety!

  - Say no if someone does something to you that you don't like or makes you uncomfortable. You are valuable and you can always say no.

  - Tell SOMEONE on your list if something bad happens. We are always here for you, and can help you figure it out.

- Check first if someone tells you that you are "supposed" to go somewhere with them and you don't know about it. Call and ask! Better to be safe by checking than sorry for getting into a bad situation!

age 15 and up

Some people think parents of children in this age group should let their children be completely independent. The fact is, your kid is a work in progress and is still testing the waters of independence. Don't throw the towel in yet. They still need your guidance and support. When children are in this age range, you need to recognize that communication can be complicated. Avoid head-on collisions. Talk gently and look for opportunities to encourage openness. Most kids don't want you to come across as the expert. Instead, they need to know you value their input. At the same time, if you don't challenge them just a little bit you may not be doing your job. They do know an awful lot and have a lot to teach you; acknowledge that and let them teach and educate you without judgment but continue to educate them—they really don't know everything and have very limited experience of the world. The lesson that there are consequences for bad decisions is very important now, especially as kids are learning to drive, so follow through and don't give in to bad behaviors. Don't be afraid to enter into an argument or two, but accept the fact that you are not going to win every one.

Boys and girls these ages may see things very differently. In general, the girls focus on taking care of others while the boys are going to be less focused on other people's feelings. What does that mean for this topic? Be aware that girls are vulnerable to being manipulated by a needy friend. Educate them about manipulation and how people can take advantage of their kindness. Seeing broad differences between genders, however, shouldn't prevent you from being attuned to personal differences. All children can be manipulated, boys no less than girls.

Kids this age gravitate toward leaders, however defined. You might not see it in your day-to-day interactions with them, but it's what they look for in friends and peer groups. Musicians, sports stars, and strong personalities, fictional or real, hold a certain appeal. Charisma and competence hold a certain appeal, too, but only if they're not coming from you. Support their pursuit of connection, but be aware of who they gravitate toward. You may not be able to dissuade them from certain heroes, but do everything to keep the lines of communication open. To reach his son, one parent I know brought out pictures of himself back when he was a follower of the Grateful Dead (a well-known '60s rock band). The point he was making was how people embrace certain groups and habits, but that these will also change over time. His son was already aware of his father's love for the band, but the old pictures stimulated a lively discussion about who the son regarded as his heroes and what interested him.

This age group can achieve great things. Ideas run wild and the sky's the limit. Yes, their brains are not fully developed and the consequences of their actions can seem unimportant to them. This is an age when they "know it all," but are clearly not quite ready to fly. They look mature, even act mature, but are not quite there yet. Today my seventeen-year-old son brought home an eight-foot couch for his six-foot room. He did not readily understand why his plan was not going to work, even if he cleared out the closet. Allow your child to problem-solve, but let him know that there are limits. Girls are still more vulnerable than boys, no matter what we think. Keep them informed without frightening them. Information is power. Empower them with what you know, but don't forget to listen carefully to what they may have already learned, and remember to tell them that you love them unconditionally.

Talking with Fifteen-Year-Olds and Older
About Safety Ground Rules

This can be a more inclusive discussion about the hows and whys of the rules.

- Who are the people who can pick you up if there is an emergency? Do you have their phone numbers? Do you know you can call any of these people if you need to?

- You are becoming more and more independent, so I want to support you and help you with that effort.

- Never go anywhere or get in a car without telling me first. We can discuss it, but you must agree to this rule. All I need to know is where you are. Why do you think I am telling you this?

- Don't go alone. Take a friend. I'm talking about safety here: Don't go meet someone you don't know alone, don't go off to a party with people you don't know. What other situations can you think of?

- You can use your judgment here, but please remember that you are valuable and that you can always say no if something or someone makes you uncomfortable.

- Please tell someone who can help you if something bad happens. We love you and can help you figure it out. Even if you are embarrassed or scared, let us know!!

- Check first if someone tells you that you are supposed to go somewhere or do something and you don't know about it. It's better to be safe by checking than sorry for getting into a bad situation!

just the facts again and again

When it comes to safety:
> practice;
>
> practice;
>
> practice!

The statistics on kidnapping and abductions are confusing. It's hard to figure out where the truth lies. Sometimes the problem is due to the way crimes are recorded; different systems ask different questions and record different data without tying it all together. Sometimes it's the way crimes are reported by the media; sensationalism sells newspapers and magazines, which encourages some news outlets to exaggerate facts, hoping to render a story even more suspenseful and lurid. Sometimes the information coming in to police departments is confusing, because too many people are involved, or witnesses are panicked and don't remember well. We know that abductions happen, and we know that children go missing and are exploited all the time. It's just hard to figure out what the numbers actually are.

Pointing out the problem with statistics is meant to set your mind at rest. Some Department of Justice statistics on child abduction report that 800,000 children under the age of eighteen go missing each year. This sounds terrifying in isolation. But if you really look at the numbers, you will come to this conclusion: Abductions by strangers are random and rare. We can also agree that even one missing kid is one too many. Spending time being on guard and anxious about the rarest kind of abduction can be paralyzing and unhelpful, just as spending time and energy on the fundamentals of keeping kids safe can make a real difference. I know for certain that communication, education, and letting kids know that they're loved can do far more than cut down on the number of missing kids and on the incidents of exploitation.

What I also know is that learning how to talk to children about difficult topics, including abduction and exploitation, can benefit your kids *and* you. Children need age-appropriate information about significant events in their neighborhoods to help them understand their parents' actions and reactions. Parents need ways to talk about difficult subjects to feel empowered and proactive. Communication—good for you and your children. Education, even about tough and uncomfortable subjects, arms everyone with the knowledge to figure things out and make better choices. And the self-confidence children get from knowing they are loved unconditionally encourages them to trust their own judgments and advocate for themselves. Learning to advocate for yourself stops the wrong people from taking advantage of you.

I hope the message you have taken from this book is that you needn't be afraid of the world, and, indeed, that I want you to see the world as a positive place. Importantly, there are things you can do to make it even safer. Remember that using common sense and listening to your intuition have a place, but so do education and sticking to the basic guidelines outlined in this book. Push past the easy answer when looking at situations. Don't be afraid to communicate with your kids. You really have nothing to lose. Use this book as a resource, and on occasion take some time to go back over what you have read. And as you reread sections (I designed it to be read quickly!) think about your own children. Where are they developmentally? What have you told them? What more can you discuss that is age-appropriate? What questions can you ask to encourage discussion? Education is power and communication is key.

Thank you for taking the time to read this book and more importantly for sharing the information it contains with your children. I hope it can help you find the words and the means to talk about some very uncomfortable topics. If just one child's life is changed for the better by this book it will have done its job. I am absolutely convinced that better outcomes start with better—wiser, informed, caring—conversations. I am absolutely convinced that together we can make a difference.

the safe kid kit

The Safe Kid Kit starts with sections I–IV. These four sections are written directly to kids and are meant specifically for them. As you will see, these sections are divided into age groups—please use the section that corresponds to your child's age as is appropriate.

Sections I–III are written to 'tweeners and teens. Section IV is written for younger kids. The same rules apply to these kids, but the information is presented in a more appropriate manner for their age group.

I want you to discuss these safety issues with your kids and make sure they understand what is expected of them. Ask questions about what they understand and what you expect and talk about it!

just for older kids

Read it alone, but be ready to talk about what you've read. Then read and sign the Safety Agreement at the end of section V.

Think about the stories you hear from one another. How many of you have been followed down the street or been scared by a "creepy" adult who seems to look at you funny? Maybe they're just weird, but it's worth thinking about, and worth doing something about, too. In a class I taught a few weeks ago, six out of twelve middle school students talked about situations in which they had been frightened by different people. Two of the situations involved being followed repeatedly by someone in a car. Here's the surprising thing: None of the kids had told any adult about what had happened. All of the kids were aware of three recent incidents in which an elementary school student had been pulled into a car. All of these children got away safely, but the point is, I know you have stories and I want you to share them with responsible adults around you. All of the kids in the class that day promised they would share their stories with a parent or other responsible adult involved in their daily life. You need to make a similar promise.

After the class was over, one of the adults who had helped set it up told me he had been molested by a teacher when he was in middle school. The teacher, whom he knew well, offered him a ride home and, during the ride, molested him. He had told only a few people about it. Now he was asking what he could do to encourage kids to speak up more, as they had in the class. He was sure it would have helped him a lot had he been able to talk about his earlier experience to someone. Even as an adult he sort of thought that the molestation had somehow been his fault in the first place. But he never talked to anyone about it and he lived with feeling responsible for many years. Don't spend a lifetime living with a dark thought; speak up.

So let's start with this: When you are walking down the street, look up. First of all, walking with your head down is just not smart; you can walk into things like cars and trees and stupid people who are not paying attention. Second, think about this: When we read about pedestrians being killed in crosswalks, we first blame the driver. And, yes, the ultimate responsibility lies with the driver. And, yes, in some cases the driver was indeed texting or otherwise not paying attention and is fully accountable. But in a few cases it has been the victims walking across the street who were distracted by texting or tuned out listening to an iPod. In California, the moment someone steps off the curb, it's the driver's responsibility not to hit them. Okay, so responsibility is clear-cut, but how much does that matter if you're the one who gets hit?

Let's switch gears. Believe it or not, forty-three percent of attempted abductions involved kids ten to fourteen. No, please don't go tell your little brother that fact; that's better left to Mom or Dad. Instead, think about awareness and staying alert in the context of abductions. There is no reason to be polite to the guy asking directions. Move away when the car slows down. Let someone else give the guy or girl directions. In my community some time ago, a male and female offered a ride to a young woman. It was really cold and rainy. I do not need to tell you the specifics of the ending, but I know it did not end well. This does not mean anyone who asks for directions is a bad guy, but why take the chance? As a kid I learned to cross the street when I saw a car parked along a country lane. It became a reflex for me, and to this day I still respond by crossing the street. And you should too.

Don't be afraid, just be aware. Be smart and keep your eyes and ears open. No, not everyone is a weird jerk, but if you can do a small number of things to avoid meeting the ones who are, why wouldn't you do them? Here's a truth: The real creepy ones don't always look real creepy. Internet lists make most of them look really old and scary, but that is just not the case. Here's another truth: There aren't that many of them out there, the weirdo couples who drive around looking for little kids, but they do really exist. Who knew?

When I first heard about the next story, I thought it made no sense, but then three different kids told me the same story! So here it is: In the mall, these good-looking guys hang out usually in pairs, sometimes in threes. They look for girls in groups. Anyway, one of them looks for the shiest one while the other guy or the two other guys kid and flirt with the other girls. The cutest guy spends time with the quietest girl, really making her feel special and then, well, things move forward as fast or as slow as they can. In one situation a girl fast-forwarded and went back to the guy's apartment and, well, did the thing she had never done before. And he took pictures. What happened next was, he called her the next day and convinced her that if she didn't love him, and do what he asked, he was going to send the pictures to her parents. She convinced herself that he loved her and really wanted her to be with him. Guess what? He had tickets to the Super Bowl. She left with him and headed to the city where the game was being played. Well, it just so happened they needed money, he really loved her, and he had a few friends who thought she was really hot. Alone, away from her parents, among strangers, the girl was trapped.

I have heard other stories that in the cities where the Super Bowl or other big sports events are held, the police get a lot of calls about runaway teenaged girls and boys. You don't usually hear these stories because the kids have supposedly never been reported missing by anybody. When they are are discovered, there is truly nowhere to send these kids because no one has reported them missing. In some cases they are from foster or other families or have moved around so much they don't have a permanent address. That part always makes me really sad. How messed up is that? People looking at what happened to these girls and boys say they disappeared 'cause they had no one to talk to, no one who really cared. But what if they did, and just didn't notice? What if you were loved all along? If your parents are having you read this book I am confident you would not be one of the unreported.

So as weird as this part sounds it has to be said. At twelve, thirteen, and fourteen you are really beginning to let go of the little kid part of you. Your body may be changing daily or perhaps it's already morphed. Things look a little different, if you know what I mean. If not, don't worry, all that is just around the corner. Here's the deal: Older guys, and yes, even girls, might just notice those changes and feel like shouting it out to you walking down the street. Most of those guys are just overgrown babies (oops! that might have been a personal opinion), but here's where our years of experience are helpful. Flattery can feel really good. I mean you think you look okay but how can you really be sure until someone lets you know? The boys or girls in your class may tell you, but in kind of an immature way. The older guys, like seniors, are really easy to talk to and kind of fun to have a crush on, but perhaps you think it's the random guys who shout out who let you know how you really rate. So those honks and "hey babies" sound really great and sometimes even pull you toward the car. Be careful here, they might not really be the nicest people. It's not worth the risk.

If you are a guy you are not in the clear. You are also at the age when attention and flattery can put you in a position you might regret later. Both girls and boys need to pay attention to older people who seem incredibly interested in spending time with them. No, I do not mean to say that they are all weird, just be aware. The bus driver who connects with you about stock cars may have other agendas when he asks you to go to a stock meet with him. What's the harm in seeing what he says when you tell him you've got to let your parents know first? If you find yourself flattered into a relationship and then uncomfortable with something that happens, speak up before it goes on too long. Sometimes older people who want to get you to do something you might not want will give you things to make you feel more mature. In one case, a fireman let boys smoke and drink with him just because he had some sick perversion about boys. Don't be afraid to tell a parent or another adult if something seems off to you about another adult's behavior, particularly if something you don't like happens. Don't be afraid that you might be wrong about a person's intentions. If you aren't comfortable, then they are doing something wrong. And if you're right about their intentions, the first thing they will try to do is block you from friends. And family. The next step is making you feel yucky about something you didn't even want to do. So if in doubt, shout it out. Talk your concerns out, and think of it as practice for when you are on your own. If someone scares you or really makes you wonder about something that you did, don't shut down, let someone in to help you sort it out. Train your parents in how to talk with you.

age 15 and up

The stupidest section of this book you will ever be glad you read.

Chances are you know most of what's in this book. Some of you have already experienced some pretty crazy, weird stuff. I bet there is even a book in a few of you, stuff your parents would never guess happened to you and yet you got through it. Some of what you've heard your parents talking about while they were reading this book probably seems pretty stupid. How many kids actually get abducted, anyway? So here's the deal, it really is important to listen up and pay attention. Really horrible, stupid, awful things can and do happen. To stay safe, information is power. No need to freak out or lock yourself in a room, but be smart, think situations through, be aware, and know the game.

Everyone knows hitchhiking is stupid. Why? Because getting in a car with a guy who pulls up next to you is asking for trouble. If you need a ride call a friend, or take a walk, but don't just get in a car with someone you don't know or know only slightly. Okay, I can hear your "well, duh" already, but there are a few things you might not know, based on stories of teenagers just like you. Kids who have been through stuff sometimes come talk to me to help get over whatever happened. Some of those kids have asked me over the years to share their stories so maybe another kid, you, won't have to go through it, too. One of the things I learned from the stories is that the most powerful way a perpetrator of hurtful behavior keeps it a secret is to shame their victim. That might seem pretty hard to do but it happens all the time. All they do is humiliate and embarrass their victim in a way that the victim never wants anyone to know about, and then they threaten to tell other people. I have had more than a few clients who were talked into letting someone take sexually explicit pictures of them only to find themselves threatened with having those pictures shown to parents or friends or posted online. Only creeps would do that? True, but you don't always know who the creeps are until later. And sometimes, when you are fifteen, sixteen, or seventeen it seems your parents are mad at you half the time anyway. Why add another level of disappointment? But, you know, most parents would rather have you tell them something like that than lose you forever. Parents tend to freak out first anyway and overreact. Give them some time and they will be okay. Yeah, I know taking pictures can be pretty sketchy, but it happens. Sometimes people can really flatter or even trick you into things you might not want to do. What too many adults get wrong is that really good kids do stupid things, and when they feel really badly about what they've done, they don't need parents adding to their guilt. (You can read that to your parents.)

I included this story in the section for younger kids, but I think it's important enough to include a version here for you. So here it is: In the mall, these good-looking guys hang out usually in pairs, sometimes in threes. They look for girls in groups, the way kids usually hang out at the mall. Anyway, one of them looks for the shiest girl while the other guy or the two other guys kid and flirt with the other girls. The cutest guy spends time with the quietest girl, really making her feel special and then, well, things move forward as fast or as slow as they can. One girl told me that things moved forward right to the guy's apartment and, well, she did the thing she had never done. And he took pictures. Called her the next day and convinced her that he was taking the pictures to her parents. It did not really bother him that he was older than eighteen because he believed she would do exactly what she did next: She freaked out, called him up, and agreed to do whatever he wanted. He said he loved her and really wanted her to be with him and, guess what, he had tickets to the Super Bowl! She left with him and headed to the city where the game was being played. Well, it just so happened they needed money, he really loved her, and he had a few friends who thought she was really hot. The game was on.

(As I said in the section for younger teens, cities where there are big sports and other events seem to have a high incidence of exploited teenaged and young adult girls and boys who have been brought there for the same purpose; and it's not to watch the game. Those girls and boys make money for whatever guy brought them there by getting paid to have sex with whatever guy will pay. You don't hear about this much because those kids were never reported missing. When they are discovered there is truly nowhere to send these kids; in some cases they are from foster or other families or have moved around so much they don't have a permanent address and haven't been reported missing. If your parents are having you read this book I am confident you would not be one of the unreported.)

Hopefully this chapter has your attention. Let's go on. So, you are a really good kid just like a girl I saw some years ago. She didn't drink, smoke pot, and certainly was not ready for sex. I worked with her for a few months in my private practice after a really bad thing happened to her, like the worst thing ever. She's okay now and I am so glad she felt okay to tell me about it, but I cannot help but wonder what would have happened if she had not told me. Anyway, she was at a soccer party with a bunch of kids. She later said she didn't see any drugs, but some of the kids were acting really stupid. She put her Coke on the kitchen counter and ran to say good-bye to a friend. A quick hug and she was back. That's all she can remember. She woke up in a room she did not know at a house she did not know feeling really confused and really lost. Her jeans were on the floor and there was sticky stuff all over her. She was really frightened and got up off a dirty, disgusting, blood-stained bed. Wandering into the hallway she saw a group of guys who pretty much ignored her. She left the house and called a friend who picked her up down the road. A few days later it went around at the high school in the next town over that six boys on the school's wrestling team had had sex with some girl that night. No one admitted who it was or what was put in the girl's drink. But my client was the girl. It took her some time to tell me what had happened. She was sure I would think it was stupid, that I would judge her; she was so upset. Before she could bring herself to talk about it, she even spoke about leaving town, only giving vague reasons until she finally 'fessed up to what had happened. I can't help but wonder how many times people disappear because of stupid things that happen to them. Something in a drink and a head full of shame can make people do really dumb things.

The stories go on and aren't always about girls. It is likely that most parents of boys aren't forcing their sons to read this book. That's unfortunate, because boys are just as much in need of safety tips as girls. So, if you're a boy and reading this, you're one of the smart ones. I think about what might have happened differently for one client, who thought he might be gay but wasn't sure. A teacher in his local private school thought he knew differently. This teacher, also the crew coach and later head of a middle school, took a group of eighth-grade boys on a camping trip every year. He figured he was "turning the boys into men." He used "tools" like exposing the boys to porn and even group masturbation. So, you might be thinking, well, this is really a rare event. And disgusting. Odds are you don't even want to think about this at all, but guess what—it can't be that rare if it keeps coming up over and over.

What does this have to do with abduction? Well, in the case of at least this one boy, what happened that year was enough to push him away from friends and family forever. In fact, many of the boys who were involved still feel detached or even estranged from their friends and families many years later due to this selfish man's actions. Were they abducted? Technically, no, but what that man did cost them years of their childhood and in some cases friends and family; so, no, it's not unlike abduction after all.

I hope you know that all those friends on your social network aren't really friends, and that the kids you're gaming with online may not all be kids but include some old guy gamer. And yeah, you would stay away from a guy like that if he pulled up in a car at night. But when you're online, it's a lot harder to figure these things out, so be smart. Protect what you say and be careful who you tell anything personal to about yourself.

I know you might not want to tell a cop, tell your parents, or reach out when something really scary happens. Your friends seem to be helpful enough, but the truth is, they are just as confused by all this stuff as you are. Speak up and let someone know when something that happened to you does not seem right. By the way, that shame isn't yours. Put it where it belongs, on the person who made you uncomfortable in the first place. Think about that for a minute. Besides, don't let it happen to someone else.

more just for kids
age 12 and up

All teens can read this section alone, but younger kids
might want to discuss it with a parent or other adult.

a word to the wise, and you are wise.

No matter how old you are, it won't hurt to pay attention to this part. I am going to keep reminding you that more wonderful than bad things happen to people. Newspapers and television often forget to tell us all the great things people do for each other. Years ago my brother was traveling around the country and lost his wallet. Someone found it on the beach, and, money and all, sent it all the way across the country to his address. He was surprised to arrive home and find it in the mailbox. Another friend lost her dog and put signs up everywhere to try and find him. She offered a $500 reward. A week later a twenty-five-year-old student brought the dog back. When she went to get her checkbook, the kid turned her down, saying he really just wanted to bring the dog home.

Remind yourself of the nice things that have been done for you.

Trust is an important part of having friends and being part of a community. Trust is something that people earn. Sometimes we think we can trust people just because they live in our town, go to our church, or serve as adults in our school. Adults can be as different as kids are. It usually takes a while to decide who you really want to share your biggest secrets with; not everyone can be trusted with who you like the most or who you think is cute. It takes a bit of time to find out who you want to lean on. We all make mistakes, like trusting a friend who blabs your story all over school. That can be really bad, because you feel like a fool, but on the other hand, with the support of your really good friends, you will recover. But when it comes to the really big things, like being "friended" by an older person who suddenly pops into your life, the stakes are much higher. Sometimes these adults can sneak onto the list of people you trust, by making friends with you and earning your confidence over time. So, can you ever believe anyone older than you? Of course, but a word to the wise: Be conscious and follow your own radar. Ask yourself if it makes sense that this adult is so focused on you. Some programs, such as mentoring centers, take very good steps to keep weirdo adults from trying to take advantage of kids. An awful lot of organizations that are there to help kids set up ways to protect kids by being very careful whom they hire. However, they cannot always screen everyone out. Even with these types of well-managed organizations it is important you pay attention to anything that makes you uncomfortable. If in doubt, check it out.

You guys know better than I do that sometimes it can feel really lonely as a kid. Parents get busy, teachers get stressed, and other adults in your life may not take the time to slow down and talk with you. The adults you get to know the best might be the people who are coaching you in sports, and some adults are just more present in your lives, perhaps more present than even your parents. Many of these people are there for the right reasons. They want to pass on something they know, or they're there in case you need to reach out to them. But that's no reason to check your judgment at the door. In my community, four coaches in the last ten years ended up in sexual "relationships" with kids. No one really wants to talk about it now because the community is pretty embarrassed. In one situation, a twenty-year-old coach molested five twelve-year-old girls. Lots of the young man's friends knew about it, but no one spoke up. In two of the other cases the girls thought they had fallen in love with their older coach, who later excused his behavior by saying that life problems forced him to make bad decisions. Being thoughtful and wise around adults just means you're being thoughtful and wise; it also means you're being safe; sometimes it really matters.

So, you have all probably been taught the notion of stranger danger. I used to use this phrase to teach kids to be aware and protect themselves from terrible things like abduction. But it turns out that's a bit of a mistake. A lot of kids think a stranger looks a certain way, that he must be ugly, mean, or just stands out in a way you'd spy immediately. But the weirdos are the easy ones to avoid. What about someone who looks familiar, like a person you already know? When the car pulls up for directions and the couple look friendly enough, why not help them out? Because you cannot judge by looks. Important rule: If the car comes close to you, step away and keep on moving. You don't need to help out. In these days lost people have lots of options like phone applications, GPS, or even 411. Why are they pulling over to ask you? They can ask at the gas station. There is no need for you to get involved. How selfish but smart does that sound?

Remember, in life there are no absolutes; things are not just black or white. You need to understand that authority figures should be respected. At the same time, remember that authority figures are as human as the next guy. You need to take care of yourself and use your judgment to discriminate rather than blindly accept their word. Perhaps that's what all those stories about the priests and others in positions of power who molested kids can teach us. Think about all those brave victims who learned to speak up. If they can ask questions and speak up, so can you!

So you knew this part was coming, feel free to roll your eyes, but please just once listen up. Most of you are on some type of social networking site. You may spend more time in cyberspace than hanging out with your live friends.

No doubt you know about not posting your address or phone number online, and not giving it out either. You have to be a little behind the times to agree to meet someone in person whom you only met on the Internet, but it happens more than you know. In plain English: Don't do it! Some percent of you will ignore this and still go. That's a dumb idea, but hear this: Tell someone where you are going or who you are going to meet. Tell your parents! Tell an adult. Okay, some percent of you will ignore this, too, but still, don't be dumb. Make a plan, and *never, ever* go alone. Finally, be smart, be wise, and pay attention to things that just don't seem right.

I'm not even going to get into sexting and sharing naked pictures of yourself because I think by now you've figured that out. Don't do it! Full stop. I constantly hear stories about how these messages and images show up online or on everyone's phones or computer without the person's permission. And don't be naïve. If you post a photo of yourself looking hot and sexy, that photo may easily end up in the hands of some sicko pervert who really thinks you're cute. Yuck! And what if he just can't stop thinking of you? How easy are you to find on Facebook or another site? He may not be able to get on your "friends" list, but he may be able to get on one of your 97,777 friends' pages; one of your "friends" who is not as wise as you, who thinks they have to "friend" everyone.

So I have covered an awful lot of material and hope you are still half listening because I'm going to say it again: The world is a rockin' place with lots of good people and good stuff going on. The odds of being pulled into a car randomly off the street are pretty slim. Family members and acquaintances commit the biggest numbers of abductions anyhow. So listen to this: If you or someone you know is going through a divorce, be a bit more alert. There are a few things to tune in to. If you hear a parent talking about quitting his job and moving away and starting to say really ugly things about the other parent, be aware. Notice I didn't say beware, I said be aware. In most cases it is fine to tell the other parent your thoughts and worries, but you can also tell a school counselor, teacher, or other safe person. If you live in a house with one parent and out of nowhere the other parent takes you away and tells you the other parent is gone, doesn't want you anymore, or has moved away, think this through carefully. Does that make sense? What if one parent told you they will hurt you if you try to reach the other parent? Please understand that if one parent takes you without the other's knowledge it's a crime. Don't worry that they might get in trouble. They need help and they need it quickly. Regardless, you should not be caught in the middle of your parents' mess. No matter how long it takes you to find a phone, tell a teacher, or tell a cop, and no, it is never too late. A parent whose children have been abducted by the other parent *never, ever* gets tired of wanting those kids back. Remember that they are there and waiting for that phone call, that knock on the door, and the biggest hug in the world.

Sometimes adults are really slow; it seems like we don't quite hear or even grasp what you guys need us to understand. Sometimes you seek out the one friend in your group whom everyone goes to for advice. If you are that adviser, consider it an honor and know you could have a great career as a therapist if you want it. As a therapist, even I need to know when I need to talk with someone who might know a little more about something than I do. Often the person we talk to is older, wiser, and more experienced. We call these people our consultants and put them on the list of people we trust (see, we have them too). If you are the one everyone turns to, talk to the people on your list when someone tells you something that makes you uncomfortable. The first part of being really wise is knowing that you don't know it all.

what's a girl to do?

You are walking down the street and a car full of "hotties" drives by and honks. If you are like I was at sixteen you might stand a little taller and high-five the friend walking next to you, but I remember that receiving that kind of attention didn't feel so good. It is one thing when you are a little older and with a group of friends, but honestly even then, when you look up and it's some thirty-year-old guy, it kind of makes you ill. Walking alone is even harder. We spoke recently to a group of seventh graders who said when someone whistled or honked when they were walking alone they did everything not to look at who it was. It scared them to make eye contact or even to acknowledge that it had occurred. One girl said it embarrassed her and she wished she could just sink into the street. A few of the girls mentioned it happened on a daily basis as they were walking home, but none of them could say what color the car was or who was in it. So here's the deal: Pay attention to wherever you are and whoever is around you. Remember: Be a Lert, the world needs more Lerts!! (For those of you who don't know, that's a quote from the writer Woody Allen. A Lert isn't a real thing but it means be ALERT.) Glance up when a car drives by and make a note of who's in it. For many girls walking alone, for some reason it feels scary or even embarrassing to look at hecklers. Fear, or a kind of shyness, pushes away a very important survival instinct, which is awareness. Of course, most people who honk, whistle, or shout are not going to pull you into their car, but honestly, if the same person or group does it repeatedly you want to know who is doing it, no? That way you can tell someone. Because it gets a little weirder and riskier when a repeating pattern occurs. So, all we are saying here is pay attention to what is going on around you. Look up, make a mental note, and talk to a parent or other adult if someone even slightly harasses you. Be alert!

On the same subject but a little different setting, I have talked to more than a few girls and boys who have told me about walking down the school hallways to rude or suggestive comments from other students. Most of the time the kids I spoke to said they took it as a compliment. A few girls acknowledged that they pretended not to hear what was said to them because they didn't know how to handle the sexual phrases. One told me she thought of it as background noise and never really listened. But one girl who had been through some very tough times as a kid told me that it really bothered her. She had a very large chest and the boys often commented loudly about it as she walked down the hall. On one particular afternoon she had had enough and stopped, looked directly at the two boys who had just heckled her, and wisely told them, "Think of me as your sister. Would you like someone to say that to her?" The boys responded with another rude comment. She did not think it had made a big difference to the boys, but she felt better because she had stuck up for herself. A million years ago when I went to high school, kids would be embarrassed to say anything like that out loud. I knew that's what many were thinking, but it was the rare one who said it out loud. Yes, times have changed and in different communities people are okay with different behaviors, but wherever you live and regardless of what is okay with others, speak up if something makes you uncomfortable.

One girl I knew made it a point in her high school to speak up if she saw senior boys making crude comments to the freshman girls. She said she noticed one girl close to tears walking down the hall. She asked the girl if she was okay and the girl had said yes, and then admitted that a few of the boys had been repeatedly harassing her for some sexual favor. She honestly did not know what to do. The older girl spoke to a few friends who helped this freshman get some of the more obnoxious boys to back off. So the message here is speak up if something makes you uncomfortable, even if it is happening to someone other than yourself.

just for the 'tweeners

Parents might want to supervise this section a little more closely. After you have both read it, ask your child what they learned, and if they have any questions or other thoughts. By asking questions afterward, you can open up a discussion about these topics and avoid any confusion or misunderstanding. You can also add some of your own thoughts. The Safety Agreement at the end of section V is for you and your 'tween to look at and to sign.

ages 9–12

This section is for your child to read alone.

I know you have learned a lot about all this safety stuff. They probably teach it to you in school and I'm pretty sure they could teach me a thing or two. So let's just go over the basics and then you can test your older brother or sister, or even your mom and dad if you want. By the way, I know that lots of kids don't have a mom and dad who take care of them. You might have a grandma or grandpa or someone else who takes care of you. When I use the words mom or dad, I mean whoever takes care of you, so you put the right name in, okay?

What do you think *being safe* means? One thing it means to me is knowing where you are all the time. If I don't know where you are and who you are with, I can't possibly be sure that you are safe. Being safe can also mean that you are taking good care of yourself and making good, healthy choices.

Would you get in the car with someone you didn't know, or someone you weren't supposed to be with? Talk to your parents about this. Why would you get in a car with that person? Who else would you go with? Would you go with someone who bought you something? Would you go with someone who was really, really nice?

Remember this: You can *never* go in a car with anyone except the people your mom and dad tell you are okay.

What if a car pulled up on the street and the man or woman driving asked you to help them? It is *very* important for you to get away from that car. You do *not* have to help. You will *not* get in trouble for walking away from the car. Even if you think you know them, they are *not* on your safe list. If you feel like you have to say something, tell your mom or dad after you have moved away from the car.

What if a car pulls up on the street and the nice people in it say they are looking for their puppy or their pet snake or their kitten? They ask you for your help. Unless they are on your list, you can *never* go and help. You will not get in trouble for going across the street to get away from them. Again, even if you think the woman looks an awful lot like your friend's mother, those people are *not* on your list and it is *not* okay to help them. You will *not* get in trouble for getting away from the car. If you are really worried about the people's pet snake, kitty, or puppy, then run home and tell your mom or dad and ask them to help the people.

If you went to the store and got separated from the person who brought you, what would you do? Think about it. Maybe you could yell the name of the person who brought you. Remember that person is looking for you, so it would help if you yelled. When you're lost and looking for your parent, no one will be mad at you for yelling in the store. You could also go to the checkout counter and tell a store employee that you got separated from the person you came in with. Sometimes kids feel embarrassed about this, but believe me, it happens to all of us! If you do this, you should wait right at the checkout counter until you see whoever brought you. Another idea would be to set up a meeting place in the store in case you get separated from the person who brought you. Do you have other ideas?

Don't always believe what people tell you. Most people in the world want to help, but if you aren't sure, then check it out with someone on your safe list. Like if someone tells you that you are "supposed" to go somewhere with them and you don't know about this, call and ask!

IV

just for the younger kids

Even though the rules are the same for younger kids as they are for the older kids, it's important to read this WITH your child to be sure that your child understands. Go slow and keep it simple!! Always check to see if your child has any questions or concerns that need to be answered. You can use this as a guideline, tailor it to your situation, and add some of your own thoughts if you would like. By the end of this section your child should have an understanding of what is expected of them to keep themselves safe. Some older eight- and nine-year-olds might benefit from reading section III (for the 'tweeners), so if you believe that would work for your child, use it instead.

A NOTE: Some kids don't have a mom and dad who take care of them. They're looked after by a grandparent or some other relative or maybe even a family friend. So whenever you see those words, please put in the name of the people who take care of the kids the most.

ages 6–9

This section was written for you and your child to read together.

Think about being safe. Do you know what *being safe* means? It means in part that your mom and dad know where you are all the time and know that you are happy.

You know there are a lot of people who care very much about you. Who are the people in your life who make you feel safe? Why do you trust them? What do you know about them?

You and the person taking care of you should make a list of these people; include phone numbers and addresses so you can get hold of them.

Would you get in the car with someone who isn't on the list of people you trust? Who else would you go with? Would you go with someone who gave you candy? Would you go with someone who was really, really nice? You probably won't ever have to think about this, but to be safe you can *never* go in a car with anyone except the people on the list, unless your mom and dad tell you that it is okay.

Now, what if a car pulled up on the street and the man or woman driving asked you to help them? It is *very* important for you to get away from that car. You do *not* have to help the man or the woman. You will *not* get in trouble for walking away from that car. You can tell your mom or dad after you get away from the car.

What if a car pulls up on the street and the nice people in it say they are looking for their puppy or their pet snake or their kitten? They ask for your help. To be safe you can *never* go and help. You will *not* get in trouble for going across the street to get away from them. If you are really worried about the people's pet snake, kitty, or puppy, then go in the house and tell your mom or dad to help the people. One little boy we know did this and when his dad went to help, the people pretended that they had never asked and said they weren't looking for their dog. So what do you think they were doing? We don't know.

If you went to the store and got separated from the person who brought you there, what would you do? Crying is good. What is even better is to stand still and yell. You could yell until the person who brought you comes. Remember, they are trying to find you too, so it would be good to yell so they can hear you. No one will be mad if you yell. What would you yell? Maybe you can make something up like in our house—we all decided to yell "Chicken Feet!" if we got separated. Talk to your parents or the person who takes care of you about this.

Another idea is to go to the checkout counter where you pay for everything and tell one of the people who are wearing a name tag that you can't find the person who brought you to the store. You should stay at the checkout counter until the person who brought you comes.

When you go to the store you need to stay with the person who brought you there and stay where that person can keep an eye on you.

What could you yell if you can't find the person who brings you to the store?

What if someone touched you in a way you didn't like, or wanted to touch you in a way that makes you uncomfortable? Do you know that it's okay to say, "No!" or "Stop, you are hurting me!"? Even though it might be hard to talk about, you should tell another adult what happened. It is not okay for anyone (kids or grown-ups) to touch you and you can say "NO!"

Practice saying "No" or "Stop it" now!

You and your child should make a list of the people to tell if someone was touching them inappropriately.

If you want to play outside you have to check with the person who is taking care of you. You may NOT go anywhere alone.

I want you to make a plan to keep yourself safe. The world is a wonderful place, but I want to be sure that you have learned some easy ways to keep yourself safe. I thought of these things for you, but you probably have some good ideas, too. What are they? Let's add them to our list of rules for safety.

ages 3–6

This section was written for you to read to your child.

Go slow and keep it simple. You could make a list of "Safety Rules" and put it up where your child can see it, even if they can't read. If you make it together, it will have more meaning for your child. Remember that children this age think that "bad" strangers look like "mean, ugly" people, so avoid using those words.

A NOTE: "Mommy" and "Daddy" are written here to represent whoever takes care of the child most of the time; substitute appropriate caregiver names as needed.

I want to teach you about being safe. Do you know what *safety* is?

What are some of the ways you could be safe?

I think *safety* means that we know where you are *all the time.* You don't ever go off by yourself without talking to me or _____ first!!

You know there are a lot of people who care about you. Who are the people in your life who you think take care of you? These are the only people who can take care of you! *Draw a picture of each person. You and your child should make a list of these people; it could include phone numbers and addresses.*

Would you get in the car with a person who isn't on your list? (I hope your child said "NO"!)

Would you go with someone who gave you candy? Would you go with someone who was really nice? (Again, your child should say "No." If not, explain why not.)

To be safe, you can never go in a car with anyone except the people on your list, unless your mom or dad tells you to!

So tell me, who can you go with in the car?

You and your child should make a list of people who are okay to go with.

If you went to the store with a person on your list and you got lost and couldn't find that person, what would you do?

You could stand still and yell. You won't get in trouble if you yell in the store.

What would you yell? Ask your mom or dad. In our house we taught the kids to shout "Chicken Feet!" if they were lost.

You always need to stay with the person who brings you to the store, and stay where that person can see you.

Make a list of what your child could yell if he or she got lost. Practice this now—it makes it fun!

If anybody touches you in a way you don't like or it hurts you, even Mommy or Daddy, what would you say to him or her?

"Stop, you are hurting me!" or even "No" are good things to say. And you need to tell one of the people on your list what happened. It would make Mommy and Daddy very proud of you if you told someone.

Practice saying "No" or "Stop it" now!

You and your child should make a list of the people to tell if someone was touching them inappropriately.

If you want to play outside you have to check with the person who is taking care of you.

You may NOT go anywhere alone.

What will you do before you go out to play alone? Talk to your mom or dad about this.

If you have other rules you would like to include, you can add them here. Do not overwhelm your child, keep it simple, and go slow!

the safety agreement

for older kids

This agreement will reinforce your expectations and rules regarding safety. You and your child can sign it together.

safety ground-rules agreement

I, _____, care about my own safety and understand that my guardian, _____, loves and cares about me, and is looking out for my best interest.

By signing the Ground-Rules Contract, I agree:

1. to keep the names and numbers of the people my guardian and I have agreed upon, in case plans change or I need someone and my guardian is not available.

2. not to go off with anyone or move from one location to another without telling _____ first. (That includes meeting someone I don't know.)

3.   not to get into a car without telling _____ first.

4.   that if I have a phone I will keep it with me at all times and will return phone calls and text messages immediately. If I don't have a phone, I will make sure _____ knows how to reach me.

5.   to say "No" if I don't like the way someone is treating me or it makes me uncomfortable.

6.   not to post identifying information, like my home address, on the Internet.

7.   to call home if I feel scared or uncomfortable, no matter where I am or what time it is. My guardian will agree to not get upset if I call them for this reason, no matter where I am or what time it is.

8.   I will check it out first if someone tells me to do something or to change a plan I have agreed upon with my guardian.

Your signature _____

Guardian's signature _____

for younger kids

This agreement is meant for younger kids and will reinforce your expectations and rules about safety.

safety ground-rules agreement

I, _____, care about my own safety and understand that my guardian, _____, loves and cares about me, and is looking out for my best interest.

By signing the Ground-Rules Contract, I agree:

1.   to keep the names and numbers of the people _____ and I have agreed upon.

2. not to go off somewhere to play by myself without telling _____ first.

3. never to go off with anyone without telling _____ first.

4. never to get into a car without telling _____ first.

5. to say "No" if I don't like the way someone is touching me or it makes me uncomfortable.

6. not to put any personal information, like my home address or my phone number, on the Internet.

Your signature _____

Guardian's signature _____

VI

safety equations

The Safety Equation is a simple way to encourage kids to assess a situation before diving in. It teaches them to stop and think for a moment and will reinforce good decision making. The skill of assessing a situation and taking appropriate action is part of critical thinking; in education and in most professions there is a call for more of this ability. The skills learned from the Safety Equation will help your child to solve problems and to figure out what to believe and what to do as they develop into mature adults.

The parts of a Safety Equation are:

- Observation: What are the facts? What do I know?
- Evaluating the evidence: Which facts are important and which are not? Is this a good, bad, or neutral situation? What could go wrong? How could I make it better?
- Taking action: What should I do? How should I respond to this situation?
- Evaluating my response: Did I make the right decision?

> Could I have made a better choice? How did my decision
> work out for me?

Work through the following examples with your children and talk together about your results. Not all the situations are about safety and not all situations are obvious, so make sure to discuss your equations together. After you read each situation, make sure to write down the answers to the questions above. You can add or subtract new details to make a situation better or worse and ask your child how the change you made affects his or her decisions. Come up with your own situations—see who can make the best equation.

Keep in mind your child's stage of development. Kids tend to be concrete thinkers and can get stuck on facts; sometimes that helps, sometimes it hurts.

6–9 years old

Situation 1: Alice and Jane are riding bicycles home from school together. They always take the same route. Today they decide to have a race. Jane takes off on her new bike, leaving Alice in the dust. Alice decides to take that shortcut she's always heard about. What's the equation for Jane? What about Alice?

- Jane: Riding home the usual route + alone + new bike = small amount of danger. (She IS alone.)
- Alice: Riding home on a new and different route + alone = potential danger. (In fact, Alice got lost and scared her mom when she came home an hour late.)

Situation 2: Sammy is playing in his room while his mom takes a nap. He hears the doorbell ring. When he peeks out the window he sees a man he doesn't know.

- Sammy: Mom is sleeping + unknown person = not a good idea to open the door. (The man will come back if it's important.)

12–15 years old

Situation 1: Olivia is going out with the "hottest" guy in the class. She is a smart girl and has a big test coming up tomorrow. Dylan wants to do well in school but he makes fun of Olivia for being a nerd. He wants her to loosen up and have some fun for once. "Let's go see a movie tonight—the late show."

- Olivia: Being a nerd + test = study for the test.
- Olivia: Being a nerd + test + pressure from boyfriend + really good movie = potentially difficult choice. (In this case, Olivia evaluated the facts and decided the test was more important.)

Situation 2: It's fifty-four degrees this morning. It's late October. Charlotte is dressed in cutoffs and a tank top. The forecast is for clouds and rain. Charlotte wants to look "cute" for the new guy she sits next to in World History class. ADD IN that Charlotte is just getting over a bad cold.

- fifty-four degrees + won't get warmer + summer clothes + cute boy = tough decision
- fifty-four degrees + won't get warmer + summer clothes + cute boy + recently sick = now the situation is more clear, the evidence to put on a sweater or jacket is hopefully stronger than the cute boy! (In this case, the cute boy won out and Charlotte ended up back in bed with a worsening cold.)

15–18 years old

Situation 1: John drives himself to a party. He is just seventeen and has a provisional license. Word is that there is an even better party in the next town. Everyone wants to go. The really hot girl from class asks if he will drive her to the party. Once they get in the car, she tells him she is just about to go for her driving test and needs some practice.

- John drives alone + provisional license = some danger (new driver).
- John drives with Suzie + provisional license + she wants to drive the car = potential danger. (Yes, John let Suzie drive and the first thing she did was knock the mirror off the side of a parked car. Luckily no one was hurt but it cost John $300 to replace the mirror.)

Situation 2: Junior wants to have "some" friends over. Unfortunately, you are out of town on a business trip. Junior thinks it's a great idea to post his address, a time, and date online and to welcome "anyone who wants to come."

- Junior + friends + no supervision = potential problem.
- Junior + friends + no supervision + online posting = definite problem! (Junior was immediately told to take the information off his social media page. Dad called a neighbor to drive by the house later that night. Junior had decided it wasn't such a great idea after all. . . .)

the safe list

This is a blank Safe List for you and your children to fill out together. You can list the names and contact information of the people on your safe list and attach a photograph, or have your child draw a picture.

_____'s **Safe List**

Name: _____

Primary Phone: _____

Secondary Phone: _____

E-mail: _____

Address: _____

_____

_____

Name: _____

Primary Phone: _____

Secondary Phone: _____

E-mail: _____

Address: _____

_____

_____

Name: _____

Primary Phone: _____

Secondary Phone: _____

E-mail: _____

Address: _____

_____

_____

Name: _____

Primary Phone: _____

Secondary Phone: _____

E-mail: _____

Address: _____

_____

_____

Name: _____

Primary Phone: _____

Secondary Phone: _____

E-mail: _____

Address: _____

_____

_____

resources and information

The resources below can be accessed for further information or help.
If you have an emergency, please call 911.

Child Abuse

Childhelp National Child Abuse Hotline: 1-800-4-A-CHILD.

 (1-800-422-4453)

http://www.childhelp.org

http://www.childwelfare.gov

http://www.safepath.org

http://www.preventchildabuse.org

Children's Legal Rights

American Bar Association (ABA): (202) 662-1720

American Civil Liberties Union—Child Rights Project: (212) 549-2500 or
    http://www.aclu.org

National Association of Counsel for Children (NACC): (888) 828-NACC
    or http://www.naccchildlaw.org

Child Sexual Exploitation or Missing Children

National Center for Missing and Exploited Children:
http://www.missingkids.com/missingkids
Missing and Exploited Children Tipline: 1-800-843-5678

Domestic Violence

National Domestic Violence Hotline: 1-800-799-SAFE (7233),
   1-800-787-3224 (TDD), or http://www.thehotline.org

Mediation and Conflict Resolution

Association of Family and Conciliation Courts: http://www.afccnet.org
Association for Conflict Resolution: http://www.acrnet.org

Mental Health

National Alliance on Mental Illness: http://www.nami.org

Parenting

National Parent Helpline: 1-855-4A-PARENT (1.855.427.2736) or http://
   www.nationalparenthelpline.org
Center for Improvement of Child Caring: (818) 980-0903 or http://www
   .ciccparenting.org

Runaways

National Runaway Switchboard: 1-800-621-4000 or http://
   www.1800runaway.org

what to do if a child is missing

In an emergency situation, it is important to know which steps to take. If you think that a child has gone missing or that a family member may have taken the child, you should:

1. Call your local law enforcement. Tell them you want to file a missing person report for an abducted child with the National Crime Information Center (NCIC). (The NCIC is the computerized database that can be used by all law enforcement nationally.) Tell them to make sure the NCIC report has a child abduction "flag" on it. Ask them to file an AMBER Alert (this is the Child Abduction Alert system and may go by different names in different states). Make sure you write down the name, badge number, or other relevant information of the person you are speaking with when you file the report. Remember that you do not need a custody order to file a report, and law enforcement

agencies are not allowed to make any delay when reporting a missing child.

2. Report a missing child using the toll-free hotline for the National Center for Missing and Exploited Children at 1-800-THE-LOST (1-800-843-5678). For more information, you can access their website: www.missingkids.com.

3. Call your local FBI field office to report a missing child. You can locate the contact information for your local FBI field office at the front of any telephone book or on their website: www.fbi.gov/contact-us.

4. Find support with the National Center of Missing and Exploited Children Team H.O.P.E. (www.teamhope.org or 1-866-305-HOPE). They can match you with parent volunteers who have experience with abduction.

5. Association of Family and Conciliation Courts "An interdisciplinary and international association of professionals dedicated to improving the lives of children and families through the resolution of family conflict" at www.afccnet.org.

If you suspect that a child has been taken across international borders, you can follow the additional steps below:

1. Access the US State Department website (www.travel. state.gov) to find information on opening a case, finding representation, and procedures by country.

2. Set up a Children's Passport Issuance Alert Program with the Department of State's Office of Children's Issues. The alert program will notify you if the passport has been used to move the child internationally. You can contact them at PreventAbduction@state.gov.

3. Find further resources and actions steps in the US

Department of Justice's Office of Juvenile Justice and
Delinquency Prevention report entitled "A Family Resource
Guide on International Parental Kidnapping." This can be
accessed at www.ncjrs.gov/pdffiles1/ojjdp/215476.pdf.

Notes

chapter 2

9 *800,000 children*: www.missingkids.com

9 "*58,000 family abductions*: http://abcnews.go.com/US/keeping-children
    -safe-stranger-abduction/story?id=14072100#.T_sqr3rnd8E

10 *The Truth about Abduction*: All statistics are from the US Department
    of Justice. Per Andrea J. Sedlak, David Finkelhor, Heather Ham-
    mer, and Dana J. Schultz. "National Estimates of Missing Children:
    An Overview" in *National Incidence Studies of Missing, Abducted,
    Runaway, and Thrownaway Children*, Washington, DC: Office of
    Juvenile Justice and Delinquency Prevention, Office of Justice Pro-
    grams, US Department of Justice, October 2002, pg. 5. The US
    Department of Justice's Office of Juvenile Justice and Delinquency
    Prevention funds ongoing research about missing children through
    the National Incidence Studies of Missing, Abducted, Runaway, and
    Thrownaway Children (NISMART). These researchers published
    their latest data in 2002, NISMART-2. The researchers will be col-
    lecting new data over the next year to use in an update to this study,

NISMART-3. To discuss the previous research, please contact Andrea Sedlak at 301-251-4211, SEDLAKA1@WESTAT.com.

chapter 3

16   *Deputy District Attorney*: Guzik, H. 4/12/2012, "Lost and Found," *Ventura County Reporter*. Retrieved 5/24/2012, from www.vcreporter. com/cms/story/detail/lost_and_found/9721/.

19   *Fortunately, there is something*: www.hcch.net/index_en.php.

22   *This is what happened in the case of*: http://www.time.com/time/ nation/article/0,8599,2030204,00.html#ixzz27EvzRbTO.

chapter 7

56   *The Maturing Brain*: Casey, BJ, RM Jones, and TA Hare. "The Adolescent Brain." Ann NY Acad Sci 1124: 111–126. 2008.

56   *as late as twenty-five!*: Walsh, D. *Why Do They Act That Way? A Survival Guide to the Adolescent Brain for You and Your Teen*. New York: Free Press, 2004.

56   *In an incident*: http://newsitem.com/news/teen-admits-to-bomb-threat -at-mount-carmel-area-1.1386414.

chapter 9

77   *girls suffer a higher risk*: 7/4/2012. RMFoundation.arsis.net.

78   *Even arranged marriages*: Stockholm, 1996.

79   *An estimated 2.5 million people*: International Labour Organization, *Forced Labour Statistics Factsheet* (2007).

79   *161 countries*: United Nations Office on Drugs and Crime, *Trafficking in Persons: Global Patterns* (Vienna, 2006).

79   *Trafficking affects*: Ibid.

79   *The majority of trafficking*: International Organization for Migration, *Counter-Trafficking Database, 78 Countries, 1999–2006* (1999).

79 *An estimated 1.2 million*: UNICEF, *UK Child Trafficking Information Sheet* (January 2003).

80 *Many trafficking victims have*: International Organization for Migration, *Counter-Trafficking Database*.

80 *Fifty-two percent of those recruiting victims*: Ibid.

80 *In Fifty-four percent of cases*: Ibid.

80 *The majority of suspects*: United Nations Office on Drugs and Crime, *Trafficking in Persons: Global Patterns* (Vienna, 2006).

Acknowledgments

This book would never have been written without the stories shared by willing families, patients, and clients. You have taught us so much about listening and really hearing. And to one particular family and individual: Your wisdom and experience have helped us understand the importance of discussing these difficult topics.

Thank you especially to Nancy Seltzer for believing in the project enough to support its conception and for being a true mentor, friend, and support. And to Mort Janklow, who believed the book was important enough to publish. And publish we did, with the incredible support of Brit Hvide and Thomas LeBien.

To our husbands: Thank you for all that you have given us. The two of you have encouraged, supported, and cheered us on throughout this process.

And last and not least is a huge thank you to our children: Chris, Chelsea, Connor, Andy, Ryan, Annie, Charlotte, and Cooper, who have taught us more than any book ever could. Each of you is well on your way to embracing your own life. We can't wait to see what happens next!

Index